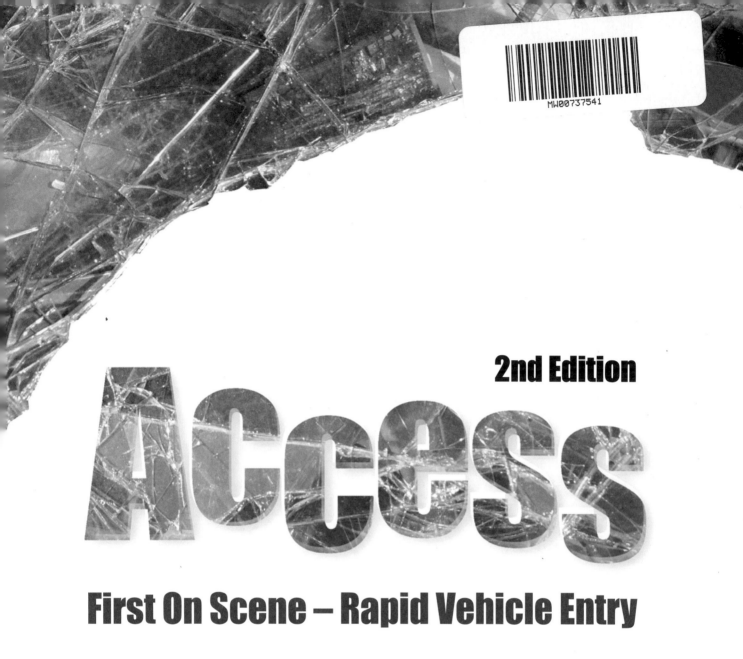

2nd Edition

Access

First On Scene – Rapid Vehicle Entry

Roy L. Alson, MD, PhD, FACEP

Wm. Bruce Patterson, Captain/EMT-P

International Trauma Life Support

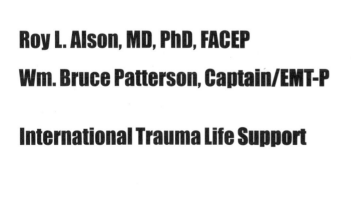

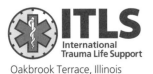

ITLS
International
Trauma Life Support

Oakbrook Terrace, Illinois

International Trauma Life Support
1 S. 280 Summit Avenue, Court B-2
Oakbrook Terrace, IL 60181
Phone: 888.495.4857
            630.495.6442 (international)
Fax: 630.495.6404
Web: www.itrauma.org
Email: info@itrauma.org

Published in the United States
by International Trauma Life Support
Oakbrook Terrace, Illinois

ISBN-10   0-9647418-4-9
ISBN-13   978-0-9647418-4-3

The information contained within this publication has been collated from several authors and has been reviewed by experts in the field of vehicle rescue to ensure its suitability for this publication. However, this publication is not intended as a substitute for the recommendations of vehicle manufacturers relevant to their specific products. International Trauma Life Support (ITLS) assumes no responsibility or liability arising from any error or omission from this publication, or from the use of any information, advice or techniques contained in this publication.

Publication Design and Cover Art by Kate McDonough

ISBN-10 0-9647418-4-9
ISBN-13 978-0-9647418-4-3

DEDICATION

This second edition of Access is dedicated to two heroes and special friends of International Trauma Life Support.

Harvey D. Grant died on January 24, 1993. Harvey will always be remembered as the father of EMS and vehicle rescue. For years, his dream was to have ambulance crews trained in quick access to accident victims, thus enhancing the usable time of the "golden hour."

James B. "Jim" Gargan died June 19, 2004, at his residence after a brief illness. Jim was considered by many to be the world's foremost authority on trench and structural collapse rescue. Jim marked his 57th anniversary in emergency services in 2004. Jim partnered with Basic Trauma Life Support International, now ITLS, in 1995, to make Harvey's concept of access to motor vehicles a reality.

ITLS thanks Barbara Gargan and her family for allowing ITLS to continue the vision.

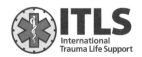

Contributors

Editors

Roy L. Alson, Ph.D, MD, FACEP
Associate Professor, Department of Emergency Medicine, Wake Forest School of Medicine; Medical Director, SMAT Program, NC Office of EMS; Medical Director, Special Operations Response Team; Medical Director, Forsyth County EMS; Commander, DMAT NC-1, National Disaster Medical System, U.S. Department of Homeland Security; Winston-Salem, North Carolina

Wm. Bruce Patterson, Capt./EMT-P
Chair, ITLS Access Committee; Captain/EMT-P, Strathcona County Emergency Services; ALS Instructor, Grant MacEwan College; Edmonton, Alberta, Canada

Contributors

Michael D. Brown, NREMT-P
Assistant Fire Chief, North Lake Tahoe Fire Protection District, Incline Village, Nevada

Anthony N. Cellitti, NREMT-P/FF
Lead EMS Instructor, Rockford Health System, Rock River Region EMS System, Rockford, Illinois

Anthony Connelly, Sr. Para., BhSc, P.G.C.E.Ed
Resuscitation Services Manager, University Hospital of North Tees, Stockton on Tees, England

Jeff W. Hinshaw, MS, PA-C, NREMT-P
Clinical Instructor, Department of Emergency Medicine, Wake Forest University School of Medicine; Rescue Operations Captain, Winston-Salem Rescue Squad; Winston-Salem, North Carolina

John Mohler, RN
Flight Nurse, Care Flight, Reno, Nevada

SSG Patrick L. Muirhead, EMT-B
Staff Sergeant, U.S. Army

Michael O'Donnell, ACP
Supervisor, Toronto Emergency Medical Services, EMS Education & Development Unit, Toronto, Ontario, Canada

William F. Pfeifer III, MD, FACS
Trauma Surgeon, Littleton-Adventist Hospital, Engelwood, Colorado

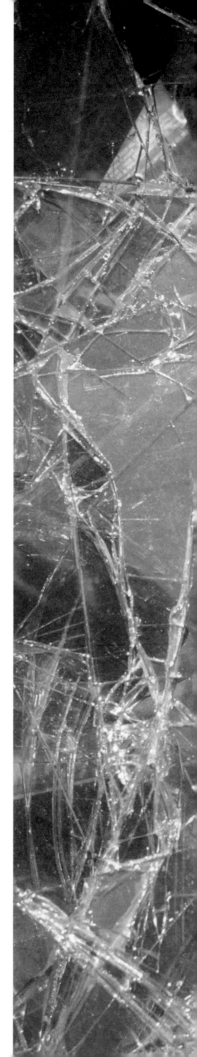

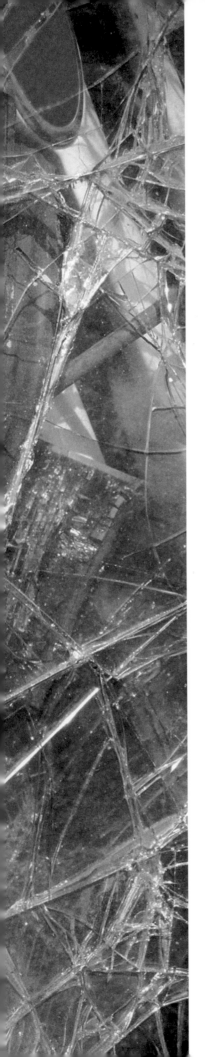

Contributors

Casey Quinlan, EMT-P
Director of ALS Education, Regional Emergency Medical Services Authority, Reno, Nevada

Vern E. Smith, EMT-P
Pennsylvania State Fire/Rescue Instructor; Basic Vehicle Rescue Instructor; Director, EMS & Police Programs, Butler County Community College, Butler, Pennsylvania

Reviewers

John E. Campbell, MD, FACEP
President, International Trauma Life Support

Donna Hastings, EMT-P
Chair, Editorial Board, International Trauma Life Support; Vice President, Health Promotion, Education and Research, Heart and Stroke Foundation of Alberta, Calgary, Alberta, Canada

Managing Editor

Kate McDonough
Communications Manager, International Trauma Life Support, Oakbrook Terrace, Illinois

Photographers

Anthony N. Cellitti, NREMT-P/FF
Lead EMS Instructor, Rockford Health System, Rock River Region EMS System, Rockford, Illinois

Sue Clemons-Tysiak
Staff Assistant, International Trauma Life Support, Oakbrook Terrace, Illinois

ITLS Leadership

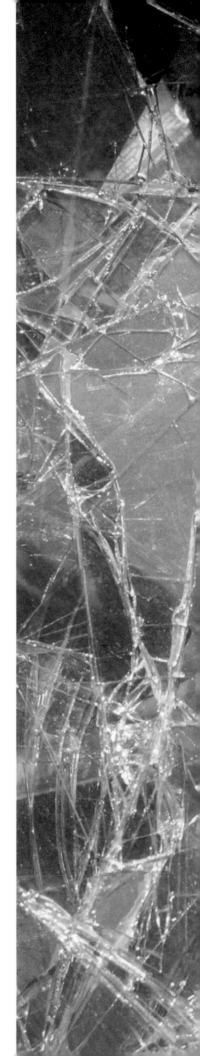

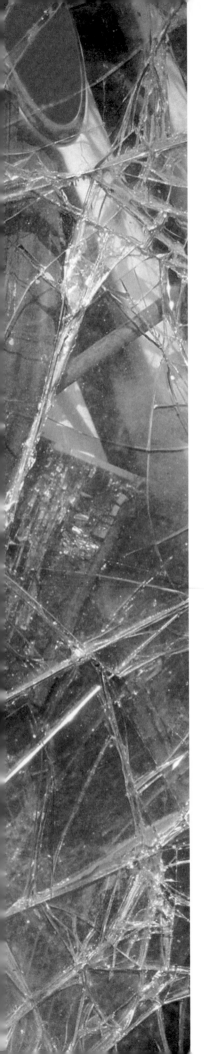

ITLS Leadership

About ITLS

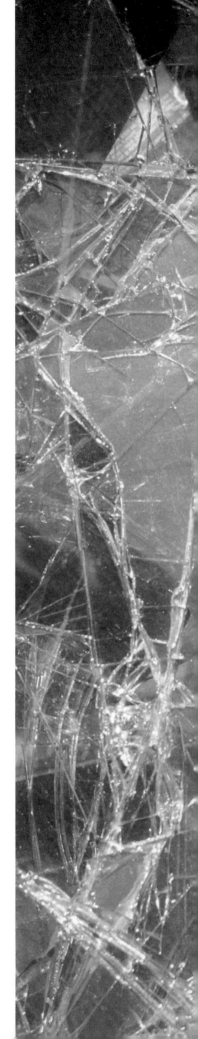

International Trauma Life Support is a global not-for-profit organization dedicated to preventing death and disability from trauma through education and emergency trauma care. Founded in 1985 as Basic Trauma Life Support, ITLS adopted its new name in 2005 to better reflect its global role and impact.

The ITLS framework is a global standard that enables providers to master the latest techniques in rapid assessment, appropriate intervention and identification of immediate life-threatening injuries. ITLS is accepted internationally as the standard training course for prehospital trauma care. It is used as a state-of-the-art continuing education course and as an essential curriculum in many paramedic, EMT, and first-responder training programs.

Today, ITLS has more than 70 chapters and training centres worldwide. Through ITLS, hundreds of thousands of trauma care professionals have learned proven techniques endorsed by the American College of Emergency Physicians and the National Association of EMS Physicians.

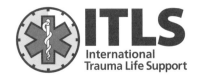

Foreword

Trauma remains a major killer, and motor vehicle collisions continue to take the lives of thousands each year. Thousands more suffer major injuries that leave them disabled. In addition to this horrible toll, the financial cost of motor vehicle trauma runs into the millions of dollars. Some reduction in the cost in lives has been made with the use of seat belts and passive restraints. Design of vehicles has improved, providing increased protection after a collision. However, those same changes that protect patients and keep them inside the vehicle also make it harder for first responders, EMS and rescue personnel to get to the patient after a collision.

Unfortunately, all too often, a first responder unit or EMS crew arrives on the scene of a motor vehicle collision only to find they are unable to reach the patient inside the vehicle. Precious minutes of that "Golden Hour" are lost, awaiting the arrival of rescue tools and personnel.

It was that "wait" and the inability of personnel to apply ITLS training that led Harvey Grant to develop the concept for this course. Harvey's untimely death prevented his completing this task. His longtime colleague and friend, Jim Gargan, picked up the "gauntlet" and came up with the Access program.

The purpose of this course is to provide first responders and EMS crews with the training to utilize tools commonly carried on an ambulance or first responder unit to reach trapped patients and begin stabilization and extrication while awaiting the arrival of rescue units. This allows us to "give back" some of the Golden Hour to the person who needs it most: the patient.

Much has changed since the release of the first edition of Access. Foremost for this book and the course that it accompanies was the passing of the author, James B. Gargan. Jim died in 2004, ending a distinguished 57-year career in the fire and emergency services. It is a fitting tribute to Jim and his commitment to the training of responders that the ITLS Access Task Force undertook the effort to update this text. We dedicate it in Jim's memory and renew our commitment to improve the care of the trauma patient by providing responders around the world with the best possible trauma training.

Numerous changes in the design and equipping of motor vehicles have transpired in the past 10 years. Additional safety devices, such as side impact airbags and the use of lighter materials to improve mileage, directly impact how we manage patients and how we stabilize and gain entry into vehicles.

What has not changed is that trauma kills. It impacts young and old and remains a major public health challenge. We do know that good prehospital care coupled with prompt transport to a trauma center or hospital capable of providing definitive care improves outcome. This course gives the first responder, EMT, paramedic or other EMS provider the basic training and knowledge to reach an entrapped patient in a motor vehicle collision and begin applying the principles of patient assessment and management taught in the ITLS course.

Trauma is a disease of time. ITLS addresses the platinum 10 minutes of the Golden Hour. There is no time to waste on the scene, as rapid transport of the trauma patient saves lives. ITLS teaches Access to help the first arriving responder gain back some of that time for the patient.

John E. Campbell, MD, FACEP
President, International Trauma Life Support

Roy Alson, MD, PhD, FACEP
Editorial Board, ITLS

Access TABLE OF CONTENTS

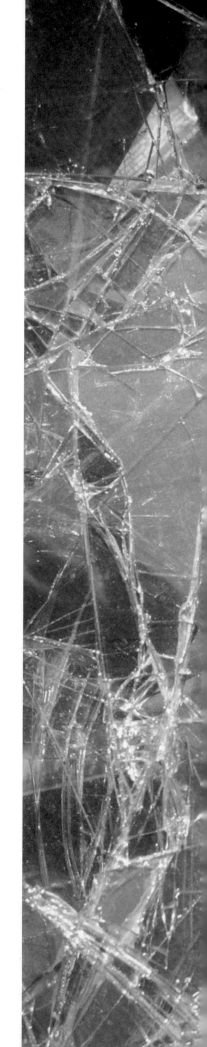

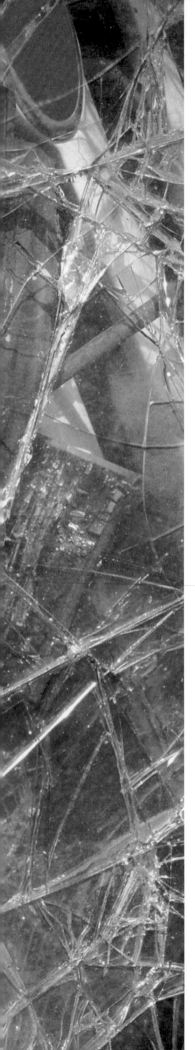

... CONTENTS

CONTENTS . . .

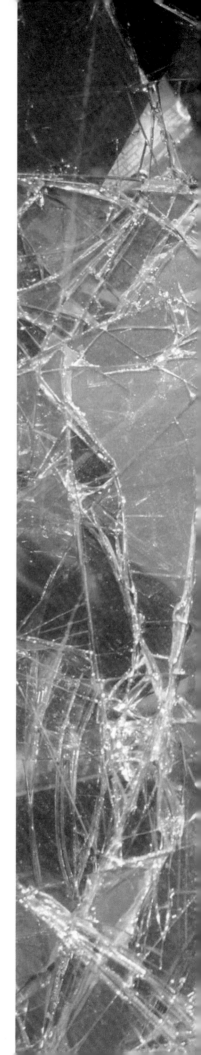

THE TOOLS TO DO THE JOB

There are specific tools needed to quickly and efficiently perform in any situation where patients are trapped. The limitations of space for storage and holding the cost to where virtually any rescue squad or ambulance service organization can afford the equipment must be considered.

The most expensive item is a portable generator (Fig. 1). The main considerations are weight, size, and amperage rating. Examples, as provided by Honda, Generac, and Coleman, are but a few available. Fifteen amp output should be the smallest considered, as this will allow the use of a tool and lighting. One 20-foot power cord with ground fault interrupter (GFI) built in needs to be "Velcro-locked" to the end of the generator (Fig. 2). Many ambulances and first response units are supplied with a power inverter allowing for 110-volt power supply.

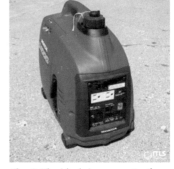

Fig. 1 The ideal size generator for a first response or ambulance vehicle.

The only power tool needed is the reciprocating saw. Both electric (110-volt and battery) and gasoline-powered saws are recommended. These should be reinforced with at least ten short (4") and long (6") blades. Be sure to buy the best blades available, such as Lenox Hackmaster 18 teeth per inch bimetal blades. New on the market are reciprocating blades designed specifically for rescue purposes. Lennox 650R and 950R are just two examples.

A few extra long-handled Allen (Hex) wrenches to fit the saws are beneficial to have on hand. It is recommended that saws purchased should not have any type of trigger lock. It can be dangerous to the inexperienced operator and serves no good purpose.

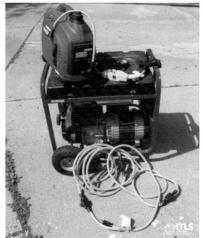

Two single tube fluorescent work lights, one 12-volt with battery alligator clips, and one 120-volt, should be carried for night work.

Fig. 2 A larger generator is commonly found on fire rescue vehicles.

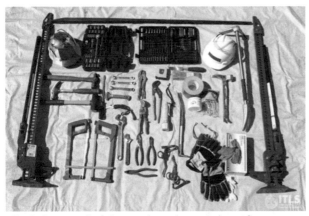

Fig. 3 Some or all of these tools can be carried on a first response unit or ambulance.

A variety of small hand tools useful during Access procedures can easily be stored on a first response unit or ambulance (Fig. 3). The tools can be stored and transported in a canvas masonry bag, the best choice because it is lightweight and flexible, or a toolbox (Fig. 4-5).

Following is a list of equipment that should be stored in the bag:

2 — Rigid frame handheld hacksaws with at least ten spare blades (Lenox Hackmaster 18 teeth per inch)
1 — 2 1/2 # machinist's hammer
1 — 16-inch large flat blade screwdriver
1 — Wonder bar (Stanley or Sears)
1 — Panel cutter
1 — Large side cutter
1 — Large (12") crescent wrench
1 — Small (6") crescent wrench

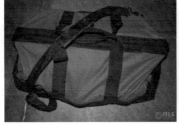
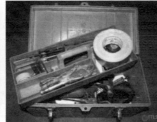

Fig. 4 (left) A canvas bag is useful for carrying tools.

Fig. 5 (right) A toolbox may also be used to store hand tools.

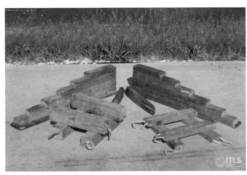
Fig. 6 Cribbing can come in a multitude of sizes and dimensions.

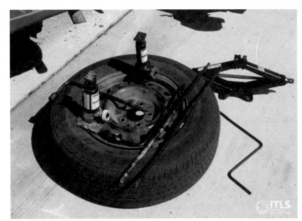
Fig. 7 Items found at the scene of a motor vehicle collision can be used for stabilization.

1 — 1/2" combination open end and box wrench
1 — 14 mm metric open end and box wrench
1 — 9/16" combination open end and box wrench
1 — 15mm metric open end and box wrench
1 — Center punch (spring loaded)
1 — Large channel lock pliers
1 — Large vise grip pliers
1 — Heavy knife (such as a buck knife)
1 — Battery pliers
1 — Battery cable puller
1 — 8' x 8' lightweight tarpaulin
1 — Roll of duct tape
1 — Box of duct seal
2 — Squirt bottles with soapy water
12 — Golf tees
10 — Cyalume hi-intensity light sticks
1 — 6' retractable tape

The following long tools are also recommended:
1 — Quik-bar or hooligan tool with pike
1 — 51" pinch bar
2 — Hi-Lift jacks

If room permits, consider step cribs or a box of cribbing (Fig. 6). This would consist of a container with 21 pieces of 2" x 4" x 18" cribbing with loops of lightweight rope stapled to the ends.

On the scene, you will be looking for (Fig. 7):
— Spare tires
— Jacks, both notch and contour style
— Jack handles

The idea is to keep the tool kit at a minimum and yet be able to accomplish all of the tasks.

Rather than trying to impose a dress code, "appropriate" head, eye and hand protection should always be worn by all personnel performing the Access procedures (Fig. 8).

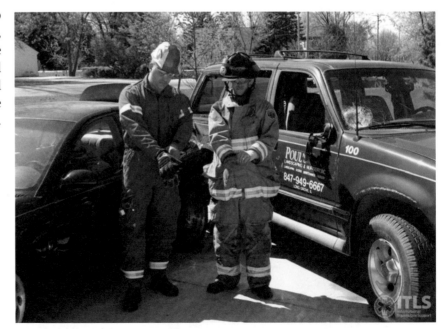
Fig. 8 Examples of appropriate personal protective equipment (PPE).

ANATOMY OF A VEHICLE

Four-Door Sedan

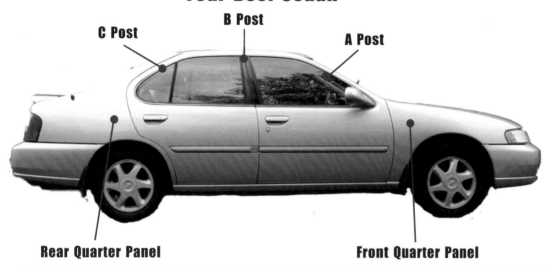

C Post

B Post

A Post

Rear Quarter Panel

Front Quarter Panel

Four-Door Sport Utility Truck

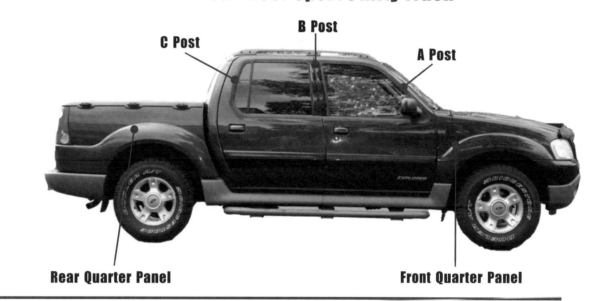

C Post

B Post

A Post

Rear Quarter Panel

Front Quarter Panel

Passenger Mini-Van

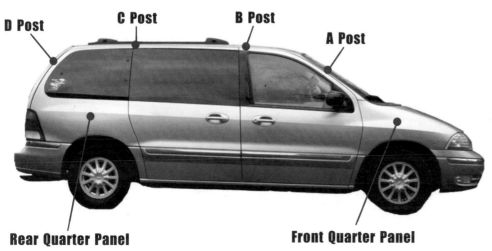

D Post

C Post

B Post

A Post

Rear Quarter Panel

Front Quarter Panel

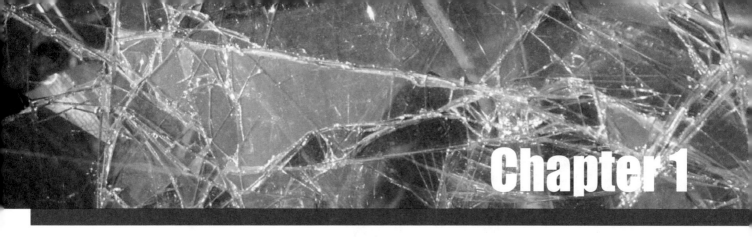

Chapter 1

Size-Up

Knowledge Objectives

The rescuer should be able to...

- Summarize activities of the size-up phase
- Determine the number of patients and perform initial triage
- List at least 10 vehicle hazards that may be present at a motor vehicle collision
- Identify an unstable vehicle
- Recognize when the situation is beyond control
- Know the operation of a supplemental restraint system
- Know the importance of identifying safety mechanisms found in newer style vehicles
- Describe the special characteristics and features of hybrid vehicles

Skill Objectives

The rescuer should be able to...

- Conduct a thorough size-up
- Stop a minor fuel leak
- Disarm the supplemental restraint system
- Recognize and disarm hybrid vehicles

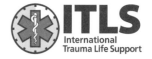

ITLS
International
Trauma Life Support

SIZE-UP

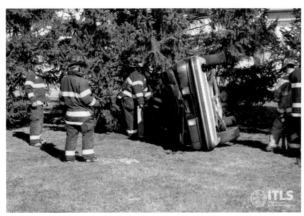

Fig. 9 Scene size-up includes a complete walk around the vehicle.

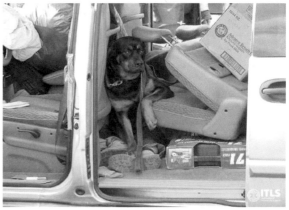

Fig. 10 A proper scene size-up will expose unexpected safety issues.

Size-up, the overall assessment of the scene, must be done in a quick and concise manner.

Look for specifics to determine what actions will need to occur. When working with a single partner, there is little time to formulate a plan or set up a command post. Yet, depending on the number of people and vehicles involved, that is exactly what may need to be done.

By conducting a walk-around, quickly determine the number of victims both in and outside of the vehicle(s), the severity of their injuries, and the hazards, if any, on or near the vehicle(s), (Fig. 9-10).

Always look inside, around, away from, and under the wrecked vehicle.

Hazards

Hazards abound at the scene of a collision. Most are caused by the collision, but some are natural and enhanced by the problem. Following are some of the more common hazards found at collision scenes.

Downed Wires

In many areas, EMTs and paramedics are not experienced in handling downed wires. End of lesson! Thou shalt not fry thy help.

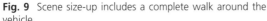

The only action is to set up warning devices (flares, lights, etc.) to avoid having someone else injured. Remember, downed power lines do not always go to ground, thus tripping the circuit. They can remain very much alive and not arcing. Always look overhead upon arrival on the collision scene. Look for dangling wires which are especially hard to see at night; a pole-mounted transformer, which may be loose if the vehicle struck the pole; and the pole itself if it snapped on impact (Fig. 11).

Fig. 11 During scene size-up, remember to look up, down, and underneath.

Pad-mounted transformers have become very popular as power lines are placed underground (Fig. 12). A vehicle can shear off a transformer and come to rest on top of it without cutting the power. This action is supposed to automatically shut down the power, but nothing is certain. During size-up check under the vehicle(s).

Do not take a chance of touching the vehicle(s) if it is sitting on a transformer. Immediately notify the power company if you are not equipped to handle the situation.

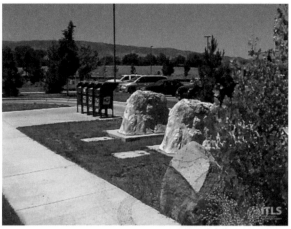

Fig. 12 Some dangers may be hidden from the viewer's sight.

Fuel Spill

If a vehicle has passed over debris or even a guardrail, there is a good chance the fuel system has been damaged.

If the fuel tank has a gash of any size, it will have dumped before you arrive on the scene. Look for a pool of gasoline or diesel fuel during size-up.

If the leak is minor, it can be stopped by pushing duct seal into the cut or puncture (Fig. 13). Be aware that vehicles may be powered by fuels other than gasoline. Propane, compressed natural gas, alcohol and electric fuel vehicles may not display the same signs of fuel leakage as conventional gas or diesel powered vehicles.

If fuel lines are pulled loose, push a golf tee or similar device as far into the rubber as possible (Fig. 14-15). Remember, if the key is still on, the electric fuel pump will continue to flow fuel if a line is broken.

Instability

A vehicle in a collision that has injured the occupant(s) must be considered unstable for possible C-spine or other injury that can be aggravated by movement of the vehicle.

Regardless of the position of the vehicle, all spring action or possible movement of the vehicle must be eliminated before the rescuers go to work on the victim. The safety of the rescuers is a prime consideration. A chapter devoted to stabilization follows.

Natural Hazards

Curbs, swales, meter boxes, hydrants, and raised flower beds are all tripping hazards that, after dark, can halt the operation by causing a sprained ankle. So be careful of your footing and always carry a light after nightfall.

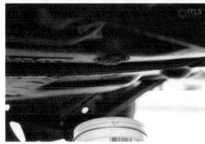
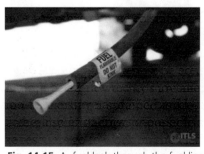
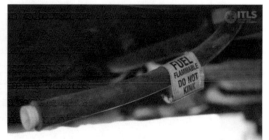

Fig. 13 Fuel leaks can be easily contained with an adhesive sealant.   **Fig. 14-15** A fuel leak through the fuel line can be occluded with a common golf tee.

Roadside drainage ditches present special problems when the vehicle rolls over and comes to rest upside down in the ditch. This action precludes entry through the doors. This situation will be discussed extensively in Chapter Four.

Creeks, rivers, lakes, ponds or other bodies of water where the vehicle may be submerged are beyond the scope of this book and will not be discussed. When confronted with this type of incident, make sure that appropriate units are dispatched to the scene.

Supplemental Restraint Systems

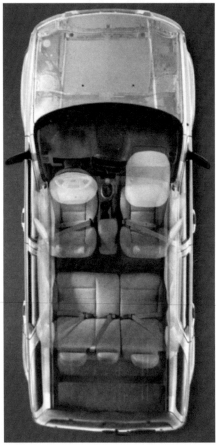

Illustration courtesy of Ford Motor Company

Fig. 16 Diagram of a SUV showing several of the 16 potential air bag locations, including driver and passenger frontal, driver and passenger front-seat side-impact, and 1st- and 2nd-row side-curtain.

Since the first edition of this text was published, great strides in passenger safety design in vehicles have been made. We must remember that systems designed to keep passengers in vehicles can also make it harder for us to get into the vehicle to care for the accident victim. Despite being a component in many vehicles for more than 15 years, air bags and other passive restraint systems continue to produce anxiety and concern among EMS and rescue personnel. Knowing how air bags operate, and their location throughout the passenger compartment, is probably the key to being comfortable with them.

We also must be aware that as vehicle designs evolve we will see more and additional types of these devices. An important point to remember is that as of publication of the second edition of this text, the number of EMS and fire personnel who have been killed or seriously injured by air bags during working extrications (in North America) is zero. Other components on the scene of the accident remain a greater threat to the health and safety of responders and victims.

Motor vehicles today are equipped with both air bags and seat belt pre-tensioners that can create problems for responders. At the publication of the 2nd edition of this text, there are 16 potential locations for air bags in passenger vehicles (Fig. 16).

Air bags can be found at the driver's steering column, below the column at the driver's knees, in the dash on the passenger's side, in the driver and passenger-side front doors, within the outer edges of the driver and passenger's front seats, in the driver and front passenger roofline/A- and C-pillar area and, for rear-seat occupants, along the outboard edges of the rear passenger seats or rear doors on both sides of the vehicle (Fig. 17-19). Other components of the system included the brain (metallic control box with capacitor often location near the driver's seat or on the transmission hump) and sensors located

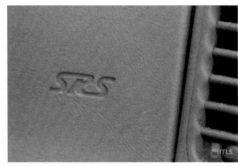

Fig. 17 The Supplemental Restraint System logo indicates the presence and location of air bags.

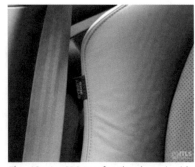

Fig. 18 An SRS tag for the thoracic side seat air bag.

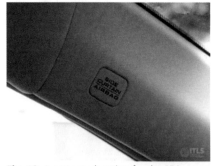

Fig. 19 A common location for the SRS stamp in vehicles with side curtain air bags.

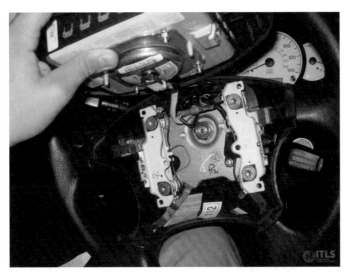

Fig. 20 The yellow wire visible in the cross-section of the steering wheel is the air bag control cable and should not be cut during accessing.

throughout the car. An important point to remember is that air bag control cables are yellow (Fig. 20). Do not cut any large yellow wires during a rescue operation.

The sudden stopping of a vehicle (in a range of 8-15 miles per hour or more) causes the forward movement of a sensor that electrically starts a burning reaction inside a hermetically sealed container, located in the center of the steering wheel (Fig. 21-23). This burning produces an inert gas (nitrogen), which in turn fills the bag(s) (Fig. 24), thus halting the forward progress of the driver and passenger — if the lap-shoulder belts are in place. All of this happens in less time than it takes to blink (1/4th of a second). Other air bag systems in the vehicle, such as passenger and side impact bags in the seat or roofline, use a cylinder of compressed gas, whose valve is opened by the computer Other air bag systems in the vehicle, such as passenger and side impact bags in the seat or roofline, use a cylinder of compressed gas, whose valve is opened by the computer, or other sensory methods. Side impact bags will inflate at a greater rate than frontal air bag systems due to the short distance between the occupant and vehicle side. Passenger side air bags inflate more slowly and with less force than steering wheel air bags, but the distance between the occupant and the vehicle is greater for these sites.

The first generation bag(s) deflate immediately. To allow for rapid unfolding and deployment of the bag, an inert powder (talcum powder and cornstarch are two of the mediums commonly used) is placed on the nylon. With activation, a cloud of dust is released. This can be an irritant and can cause bronchospasm, especially in asthmatics. Many people may believe the car is on fire, but in reality it is the gas being released from the bag that mimics smoke from the passenger compartment. Minute particles of a slightly alkaline powder may be present as a by-product of the sodium azide used to produce the gas. This could cause a minor caustic burn or allergic reaction.

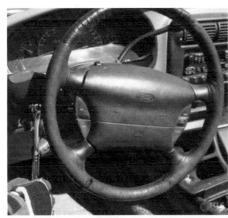

Fig. 21 Always consider the possibility of dual stage airbags.

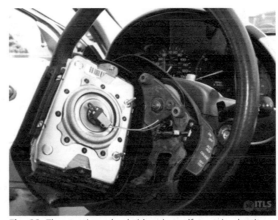

Fig. 22 The steering wheel airbag is a self-contained unit.

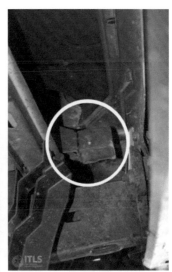

Fig. 23 An airbag deployment sensor found in the front bumper.

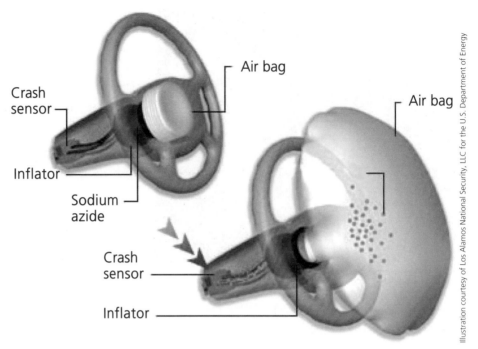

Crash sensor

Air bag

Inflator

Sodium azide

Air bag

Crash sensor

Inflator

Illustration courtesy of Los Alamos National Security, LLC for the U.S. Department of Energy

Fig. 24 Diagram of the electrical and chemical reaction that take place during airbag deployment.

Second generation air bags, also known as 'smart air bags' have multiple capabilities. Sensors placed in the seats allow the brain of the system to know the size of the occupant in the seat or even if the seat is occupied, the direction of impact, and if the victim is in position to have the airbag deploy accordingly. Most smart air bags have a split charge (dual stage) that allows a partial inflation for smaller occupants and a double charge for larger occupants. In a collision the larger charge may deploy and the smaller charge remain intact (for a second collision) and be of concern to the rescuer, in that despite being deployed, the bag can fire a second time.

Studies show injuries attributed to air bags range from abrasions to cervical fractures, apparently from hyperextention. Most serious injuries were to occupants who were not restrained by lap-shoulder belts. The bag is designed to be most effective, when the occupant is in the correct position, which is maintained by the seat belt. Other air bag-related injuries include abrasions and blunt face trauma. It is important to emphasize that rear facing child seats should never be used in the front passenger seat that has an air bag, due to risk of death of the infant, should the bag deploy.

Classically we have been taught that a "spider" in the windshield signifies that an occupant has struck the windshield. With some passenger side air bags, which bounce off the windshield, a linear spider pattern may be seen, due to impact of the cover. Spidering on the driver's side is always indicative of an occupant impact.

Following a collision, if the air bag does not deploy, as in a side or rear collision, simply disarm the system by disconnecting the negative (black) cable on the vehicle's battery. The capacitors used to fire the system will drain off in a short amount of time (ranges from seconds to just a few minutes). Do not delay the rescue/treatment effort; just work around the bag area. Chances of an accidental deployment are nil. Since 1991 when air bags were introduced as standard equipment on North American vehicles, only 5 rescuers have been injured in 3 incidents involving an undeployed air bag on the scene of an accident. A good rule of thumb is the *5-10-20 rule*. Stay at least 5" away from a side impact bag, 10" away from a steering wheel bag, and 20" away from a front passenger bag. A number of systems are marketed to try to contain undeployed air bags should they accidentally fire during a rescue. These devices increase the time needed to extricate the injured victims and their effectiveness remains unproven.

Head protection systems are becoming more common with 50% of cars in 2006 having this air bag option. These head systems utilize a stored gas inflator to function during an accident. The inflated curtains offer additional protection in rollover accidents (some last up to 3 complete rolls of the car or 5 seconds) and are even larger than passenger front air bags. As much as these bags provide additional protection, they also create additional hazards for the rescuer. The canister used in the system is pressurized to 4500 psi and can be easily cut thru with most any rescue tool. The canisters are typically stored in the middle or bottom of the "A" pillar or "C" pillar of the roof.

This means the days of a rescuer cutting and prying anywhere on a car to force entry are now over. Rescuers must identify the location of these additional SRS modules and components before the access procedures begin. One suggestion is to use the "peel and peek" method. Use a screwdriver or wonder bar to peel away the plastic on the posts in an attempt to locate these SRS components. One should also look in the B pillar for seat belt pre-tensioners, which use a small burning charge, usually nitrocellulose, to tighten the seat belt against the occupant.

There are other types of air bags either in production or being considered for production. Some of these include knee bolster bags and seat tilt bags (to prevent submarine type injuries), carpet bags (to reduce foot, ankle and lower leg injuries), along with bumper and windshield bags for pedestrian accidents.

Air Bag Scanning

The scanning for air bag identifications allows the rescuer to follow a systematic method of looking for and locating air bag identifications as well as the individual air bags themselves. This technique allows the responding rescuer to survey the vehicle without fear of missing any critical identifications in the process.

Air bag scanning begins after it is determined that it is safe to work around, touch and enter the crashed vehicle. Upon completion, you should report your findings on the presence of air bags, their locations and their deployed or loaded status to the crew leader or other supervisor.

The sequence presented here is for a typical four-door sedan situated on level ground. Once you become comfortable with air bag scanning, the procedure can be applied to other types of vehicles. Practice this scanning sequence until you can assure yourself that you are systematically looking at all possible air bag ID locations. Once comfortable and proficient in this process, full front and rear scanning should be completed within 30 seconds.

Procedure for Air Bag Scanning
Front and Roofline

1. **Approach the vehicle from the driver's side:**

    a. Open driver's front door.

    b. Inspect edge of driver's door near latch mechanism for factory-applied adhesive air bag system decals.

   c.   Inspect inside of door trim panels along armrest for "SRS" letters imprinted in material (door-mounted side-impact air bags).

   d.   Visually scan outside edge of seatback, starting at top headrest area and scanning to bottom hinge area (seat-mounted side-impact air bags).

   e.   Scan lower edge of seat cushion and seat trim material beginning at hinge and progressing to front edge of seat.

   f.   Scan along rocker channel (panel) and seat-adjustment track from front of seat edge back toward base of B-pillar.

   g.   Scan B-pillar from bottom to roofline with special attention near latch/lock mechanism (adhesive air bag decals).

   h.   Scan across vehicle to inside trim at top of A-pillar on opposite side of vehicle.

   i.   Scan from passenger's side to driver's side across dashboard and steering column (dual front driver and passenger air bags).

   j.   At driver's instrument panel, look below column for possible knee air bag system.

   k.   Scan along driver's side of dash along base of windshield area until VIN plate is located at base of left A-pillar.

   l.   Scan VIN plate for air bag ID (SRS ID near VIN plate or small windshield decal).

   m.   Note any deployed or loaded air bags discovered during scanning. IF A BAG IS DEPLOYED, QUICKLY SCAN THE BAG FOR NOTATION OF WHETHER IT IS A DUAL STAGE BAG.

Rear

2. Move to rear door on the driver's side of the vehicle:

   a.   Open rear door, if possible.

   b.   Inspect edge of door near latch mechanism (side-impact air bag IDs).

   c.   Inspect inside of door trim panels along armrest for SRS letters imprinted in material.

   d.   Scan outside edge of seatback, starting at top and scanning to bottom hinge area (side-impact air bag IDs).

   e.   Scan lower edge of seat cushion and seat trim material beginning at hinge and progressing to front edge.

   f.   Scan along rocker channel (panel) from front of seat edge toward base of C-pillar.

   g.   Scan C-pillar from bottom to roofline with special attention near rear door latch/lock mechanism.

   h.   Note any deployed or loaded air bags discovered during scanning.

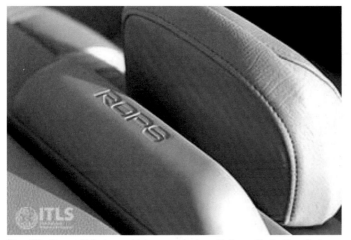

Fig. 25 Convertible-top vehicles may feature Rollover Protection System, identified by a ROPS imprint typically located near the headrests.

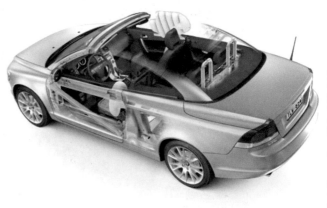

Fig. 26 A diagram of the components that comprise a convertible-top vehicle's Rollover Protection System.

Illustration courtesy of Volvo Public Relations

Additional Passenger Safety Mechanisms

- Obscure or hidden rollover protection in sedans with convertible tops (Fig. 25-26)

- Gas shock absorber bumpers on front and rear of vehicle

- Gas shock absorber on tail gates and hoods of vehicles:
    - SAFETY TIP: When under pressure, fire can cause shock absorbers to explode and produce a projectile from the internal rod.
    - If cut with tools, fluid will release under high pressure.

Hybrid Vehicles

A hybrid vehicle uses multiple propulsion systems to provide motive power. "Hybrid" most commonly refers to gasoline-electric hybrid vehicles which use gasoline (petrol) and electric batteries for the energy used to power internal-combustion engines and electric motors (Fig. 27). Any vehicle is a hybrid when it combines two or more sources of power that can directly or indirectly provide propulsion power; the gasoline-electric hybrid car is just that — a cross between a gasoline-powered car and an electric car.

Rescue teams are concerned about these vehicles because they present unfamiliar challenges at the scene of a collision. Among these is the potential for an electric motor that is inadvertently left on to move the vehicle during a rescue operation or the risk of electrical shock.

With a hybrid vehicle, responders cannot easily determine that a quiet-running electric power train is entirely shut down, compared to a gasoline-powered engine. This raises the possibility a hybrid might suddenly lurch ahead or that high-voltage wires might be cut in a fast-paced rescue. Although the procedure for disarming this type of vehicle could be as simple as opening the car door and

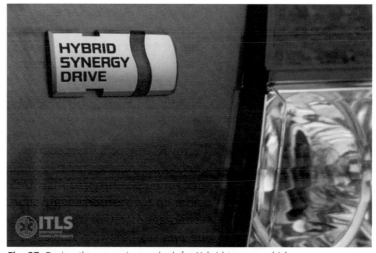

Fig. 27 During the scene size-up, look for Hybrid tags on vehicles.

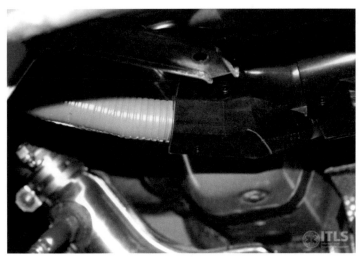

Fig. 28 Always be aware of HVS (high-voltage system) lines, easily recognizable by the orange shielding covering the wires in many hybrid vehicles.

pressing a button marked "power" on the dashboard, each hybrid manufacturer has unique differences. In most instances, rescuers must check for a "ready" light on the dashboard (which indicates the car is on) before pushing the power button to turn it off.

A more effective method requires opening the rear hatch, removing the luggage compartment floor and reaching to disconnect the car's 12-volt battery which isolates the power systems. But even then — this is a warning — the high-voltage system can hold a charge for a few extra minutes.

Fortunately, in many cases the high-voltage circuits in today's hybrids can be easily recognized by orange shielding covering the wires. This is a convention among automakers and should become an industry standard (Fig. 28).

In some hybrid models there is a removable circuit breaker mounted next to the high-voltage battery. A rescuer wearing electrical safety gloves can remove it to disable the system. In others, you can find a service disconnect switch panel or shutoffs that look like light switches near the rear seat backs or in the center of the cargo area.

One last note: some vehicles are equipped with ignition locks that do not require a mechanical key (Fig. 29). They rely on coded radio signals from a small transmitter to secure the car. This transmitter could be difficult to find, since it may in the driver's pocket rather than in a dashboard slot. If the remote key is in the driver's pocket, it will activate the car within 16 feet of the receiver in the car. It is imperative to keep the victim or the key fob away from the accident

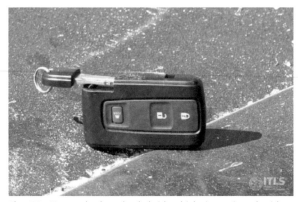

Fig. 29 Note whether the hybrid vehicle is equipped with a "smart key," and anticipate the potential hazards associated with this remote key.

site to reduce the chance of the engine becoming active when it senses the presence of the key fob.

Within this wide range of possibilities, the only sure way to approach this issue is for responders to have specialized training to help them address the new challenges. Responders should always keep in mind that a hazard is something that can affect you when you are uneducated or unprepared.

Good sources of information are the emergency response guides that many car manufacturers have published on their web sites or make available from their local dealers. These guides are considered the best source of information because the manufacturers can provide diagrams of wiring paths, locations of cut-off switches, and guidance on the best ways to extricate victims safely from these vehicles.

Alternative Fuel Vehicles

Another potential source of danger for the rescuer is the motor vehicle accident involving an alternative fuel vehicle (AFV). There are five common types AFV:

- Liquefied petroleum gas
- Compressed natural gas
- Methanol
- Ethanol
- Electric

The first priority when responding to a motor vehicle collision is to distinguish alternative-fueled vehicle from standard fueled vehicles. Look for special fuel ports, distinctive profiles, and any written markings on the vehicle. Unfortunately, there currently is not a standard marking system (symbol, logo, or placard) for these new type vehicles. One potential clue can be noted by the type of vehicle itself. The majority of AFV vehicles are part of "fleets" operated by such businesses as bus companies, taxi companies, or utility provider companies. When performing the visual size-up of the accident, the fuel containers for AFVs will most often be found in one of four locations:

- Trunk area
- Side panel of a van or bus
- Frame rail
- Pickup truck bed

Compressed Natural Gas and Liquefied Petroleum Gas Vehicle Incidents

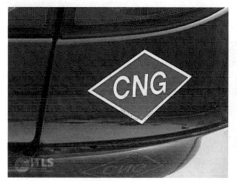 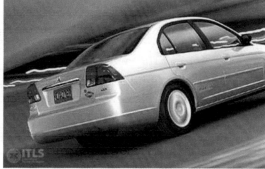

Fig. 30-31 CNG vehicles may be identified with a diamond-shaped logo placed on the rear bumper, but rescuers should be aware that such markings are not mandatory. Inspecting the gas tank will provide more information.

Traditional rescue techniques still apply when responding to collisions involving AFVs. If the vehicle is not on fire and no obvious leak is detected, stabilize and secure the vehicle by your agency's predetermined methods (setting the brake, utilizing wheel chocks, or cribbing as needed). Once the vehicle is stabilized, turn off the vehicle's ignition and turn the gas cylinder valve handle to the "off" position.

If the vehicle is on fire or a leak is detected, do not approach the vehicle. Secure the scene and provide a safety working zone with non-pyrotechnic traffic devices such as cones. Do not use flares.

Approaching the CNG (Fig. 30-31) or LPG (Fig. 32) vehicle that is leaking fuel or on fire should only be attempted when wearing proper

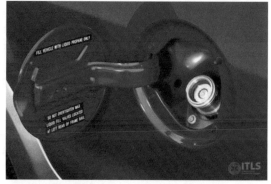

Fig. 32 The inside of the gas cap reveals that this vehicle requires Liquefied Petroleum Gas as fuel.

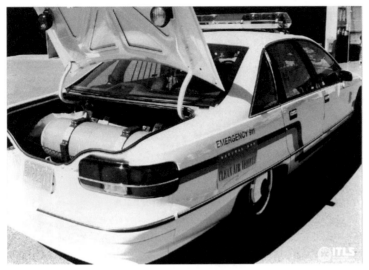

Fig. 33 In this CNG-fueled police car, the compressed gas fuel container is located in the trunk of the vehicle.

protective equipment and self-contained breathing apparatus. If you do not have the proper protective gear, equipment and training to deal with fire or hazardous materials emergencies, do not approach the vehicle. Fortunately, in most cases, an alternative-fueled vehicle in a crash should not require a hazardous materials response.

The greatest hazard of the compressed gas containers (Fig. 33) exposed to fire or extreme heat is BLEVE (boiling liquid/expanding vapor explosion) which results in catastrophic failure of the container with severe damage to the surrounding area.

When compressed gas fuel containers become compromised, the fuel converts from a liquid to a vapor that could rapidly produce a sizeable vapor cloud which may ignite and flash back to the fuel source.

Methanol and Ethanol Vehicle Incidents

Both methanol and ethanol are used in the vehicle's existing fuel tanks so there will not be a separate gas container on the vehicle (Fig. 34-35).

If there is no fire or leak, carefully approach the vehicle, turn off the driver's ignition switch and stabilize the vehicle by methods used by your agency (parking brake, wheel chocks, cribbing).

If fire is present, stay away from the vehicle, secure the area and prevent other responders from entering the area. Remember that a fire fueled by methanol or ethanol burns bright blue and can be difficult or even impossible to see on a clear day. If you do not have the proper protective gear, equipment or training to deal with fire or hazardous materials emergencies, do not approach the vehicle.

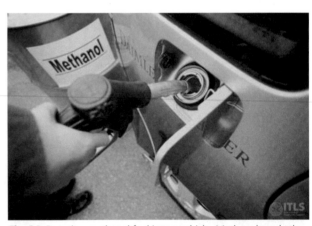

Fig. 34 Pumping methanol fuel into a vehicle. Methanol- and ethanol-fueled vehicles do not require a separate gas container on the vehicle, as they use the existing gas tank.

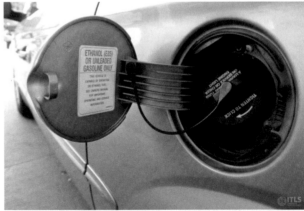

Fig. 35 The vehicle's capability to run on ethanol fuel is noted on the inside of the gas cap.

Electric Vehicle Incidents

During your visual scene assessment, look for an electric charging port on the side or front of the vehicle, the electric logo, or a distinctive profile (Fig. 36-38). These vehicles are powered by batteries, as high as 300 volts, usually located under the hood, in the trunk, or under the vehicle. A traditional 12 volt battery is still needed to operate the vehicle's electric features and will be located in a separate location from the larger battery unit. Another unique feature of electric vehicles is that all high voltage wiring and connectors are bright orange. Never handle any orange wiring, or the orange components attached to it.

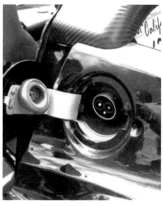 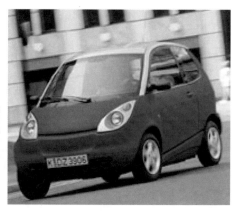

Fig. 36 The charging port of an electric vehicle is usually located on the side or the front of the vehicle.

Fig. 37 The compact shape of this European-made electric car, Th!nk Nordic's City, is typical of electric vehicles, making them easily recognizable.

If there is no fire or battery liquid leak, carefully approach the vehicle, turn off the driver's off/on switch, and stabilize the vehicle using traditional methods (set the parking brake, use wheel chocks, or use cribbing to secure the vehicle). If smoke is visible, no one should approach the vehicle without self-contained breathing apparatus. Toxic fumes and vapors from damaged batteries can be carried in the smoke or steam. Remember that all high voltage batteries contain potassium hydroxide solution with a pH of 13.5, which is highly alkaline and can result in severe injuries to the skin and mucous membranes.

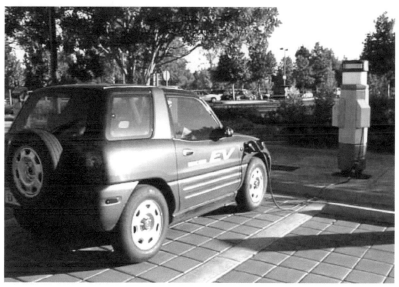

Fig. 38 The Toyota RAV4-EV, discontinued in spring of 2003, sports the distinctive Electric Vehicle logo. Charging stations where electric vehicles can be plugged in and recharged are available in some cities, primarily in Europe.

Never cut into the battery pack or the traction cable, even if the high voltage has been shut down, because the battery pack can remain charged. Since there still may be toxic fumes present around the vehicle after the fire is contained, only those with proper protective gear, equipment and training should participate in the cleanup.

Many of the models currently in production also have a "sleep mode". The gasoline engine will shut off when the vehicle stops in traffic (i.e., waiting at a stop light). If the accelerator is depressed, the electric motor instantly powers the drive wheels while the gasoline engine remains off. Stabilizing the vehicle and chocking the wheels to prevent forward motion is a critical safety maneuver for electric vehicle accidents. Rescuers should move the gear selector into the "park" or "P" position and turn the ignition key to the "off" position.

Manufacturers of alternative-fuel and hybrid vehicles have developed emergency response guides that are available online and in hard copy.

Accident Victims

Identifying the number of victims in a collision is one of the most important functions of size-up. A good survey of the scene will show how many persons are supposed to be in the vehicle(s). Note the words "supposed to be." Victims could be ejected in a roll-over, walk away from the scene, or be hidden by the wreckage.

If no one is conscious upon arrival at the scene, try to determine the number of victims by looking for clues such as school books or backpacks but no children, or three briefcases but only two people in the car. Look for clues that do not add up. Be suspicious.

This is triage time! Although a drunken driver pinned behind the wheel may be bleeding profusely and wailing like a baby, cuts may be superficial. Beware of the non-speaking person staring straight ahead and saying nothing. Triage victims using the ITLS Primary Survey (see Fig. 112 on Page 47) to identify critical life threats.

Key Points to Remember

- Specifics of vehicle design will vary between car manufacturers, such as:
  o Location of the fuel tank
  o Type of fuel pump-mechanical vs. electric
  o Door latch mechanisms
  o Hinges - cast vs. pressed
  o Location of batteries
  o Uni-body vs. frame

  It is important to familiarize yourself with the basics of vehicle design, which change regularly

- Do not use "Silly Putty," modeling clay, or any petroleum-based product that will dissolve in gasoline.

- Supplemental restraint systems (air bags):
  o Powder on surface of the air bag(s) is either talc or cornstarch. It is harmless.
  o The amount of sodium azide in the sealed canister is only 90 grams. It cannot leak out.
  o During deployment, the sodium azide is consumed.
  o Inflation is to a pressure of 4 psi
  o Multiple locations of air bags

- Hazard control is extremely important:
  o Be aware of your surroundings.
  o Do not assume someone else is going to correct the problem.
  o Always think of downed wires as LIVE!
  o Look up, around and under the vehicle.
  o Roadside ditches can be "highways" for wildlife such as snakes and alligators.
  o Immersion in water increases the risk of hypothermia in both victims and rescuers.
  o Flowing water could easily sweep away victims and rescuers.

o   Never wade into unknown water unless tethered to a lifeline.

■ Victims can be anywhere:
o   If victim is conscious, ask if anyone else is involved.
o   Look for clues that victims may have wandered off: footprints in snow or mud, crushed weeds or broken branches.
o   Look for clues that could indicate the presence of other passengers (coats, toys, child car seats).
o   Check glove and other compartments for identification materials.

■ Alternative Fuel Vehicle (AFV) incidents:
o   Identify the alternative fuel vehicle by its special markings and equipment. Since most vehicles are modified, the Vehicle Identification Code (VIN) will not help identify the vehicle.
o   When approaching or working around any alternative fuel vehicle, first stabilize and secure it by setting the brakes and utilizing wheel chocks or other forms of cribbing, especially if the vehicle is upside down or on its side. Turn off the ignition.
o   Alternative fuel emergencies require non-pyrotechnic items such as cones to secure the scene. DO NOT USE FLARES!
o   Methanol and ethanol may burn bright blue and the flames may be almost invisible on a clear day.
o   When approaching electric vehicles, be aware of toxic vapors, gases, and fumes, even after a fire is extinguished.
o   Emergency personnel should participate in prevention programs in the community. For example, if a company has a fleet of alternative-fueled vehicles, encourage them to understand these issues.

Text related to alternative fuel vehicles and AFV safety and extrication procedures has been adapted for use by ITLS with the permission of the U.S. National Highway Traffic Safety Administration (NHTSA). NHTSA maintains that the emergency response guides provided by the manufacturers are the best source of detailed information related to alternative fuel vehicles, as the manufacturer can supply diagrams of wiring paths, locations of cut-off switches, and guidance on the best ways to extricate occupants safely from these vehicles.

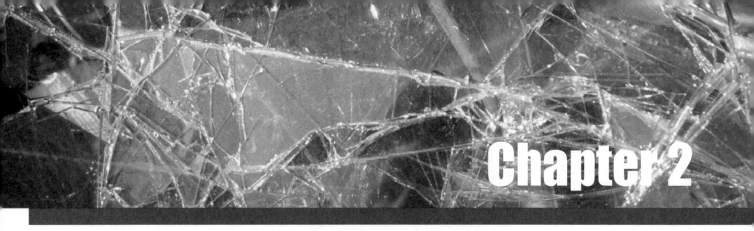

Chapter 2

Call for Help and Set-Up

Knowledge Objectives

The rescuer should be able to...

- Determine the exact location of the collision scene
- List the tools needed to accomplish the rescue
- Know and describe where to place the tools

Skill Objectives

The rescuer should be able to...

- Report the exact location of the collision scene
- Set up the equipment needed
- Gather additional devices needed for stabilization

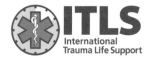

ITLS
International
Trauma Life Support

CALL FOR HELP AND SET-UP

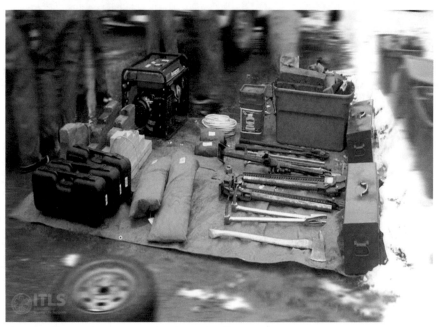

Fig. 39 Taking a minute to organize the tools will save time.

Call for Help

Barring any unforeseen circumstances, the size-up should take seconds rather than minutes. If the rescuer does not have a portable radio, the first act upon returning to the vehicle should be communication with the dispatcher. This may be the last communication until the victim is extricated. The most important message to the dispatcher is your final and exact location.

A brief summary of the number of victims and their entrapment problems along with requests for support equipment should be the extent of communication. Remember, stabilization of the vehicle(s) and the primary survey of the victim(s) are top priority.

If portable communications are available, a more detailed account can be relayed after the priorities are addressed.

Setting up the equipment is next.

Setting Up

Spread the tarp on the ground. To secure the tarp, place the generator, Quik Bar, Hi-Lift jack and other equipment on the four corners.

Place the contents of the canvas bag discussed earlier directly in the center of the tarp (Fig. 39).

Laying out the tools will make it easier and safer to find the tool of choice. This will also avoid groping in the bag blindly and possibly getting stuck or cut by a sharp tool. If a tool box is used in place of the masonry bag, take the top shelf of the tool kit and place it beside the box. This will allow visualization of tools located in both parts of the box.

This action should be done within ten feet of the vehicle to be entered. Allow enough room to remove doors or drop the side without setting up a tripping hazard.

All tools must be returned to the tarp after use to avoid losing them in grass or having them kicked under debris or the vehicle. Long tools, cribbing or any tools not being used should be kept on the tarp at all times.

Depending upon stabilization needs, while one rescuer sets up the tool depot, the other crew member can gather stabilization devices such as jacks (both notch style and contour style), jack handles, scissor jacks, hub caps and spare tires. These could be from the vehicle involved in the collision, other passing cars, police cars or even the ambulance.

Key Points to Remember

- Call for help should include:
    - Number of victims
    - Condition of victims
    - Exact location of the collision
    - Specific hazards
    - Additional help needed for patient care, rescue and hazards
    - Safest route to the scene and staging location, if any

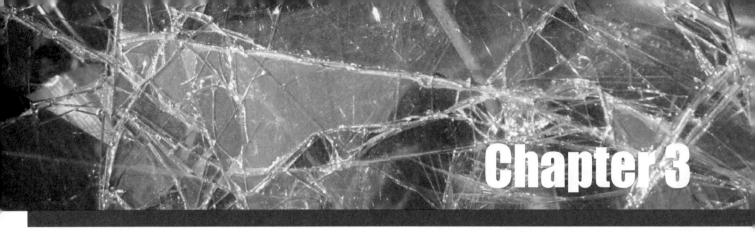

Chapter 3

Vehicle Stabilization

Knowledge Objectives

The rescuer should be able to...

- List the positions in which a vehicle is unstable
- Describe the stabilization process

Skill Objectives

The rescuer should be able to...

- Stabilize a vehicle on its wheels
- Stabilize a vehicle on its roof
- Stabilize a vehicle on its side
- Stabilize a vehicle temporarily with improvised materials, such as a spare tire

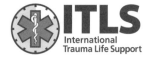

ITLS
International
Trauma Life Support

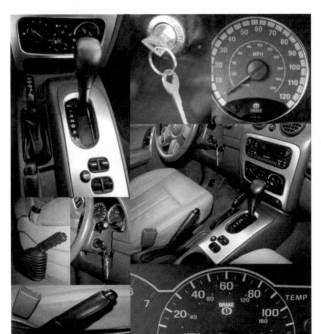

Fig. 40 Always consider the steps to make the scene safe.

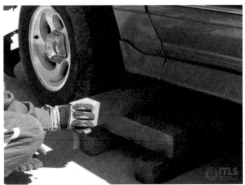

Fig. 41 Assure proper positioning of cribbing. Example for an "A" pillar stabilization.

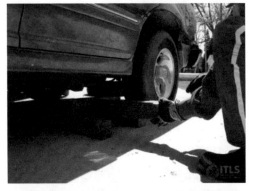

Fig. 42 Example for a "C" pillar stabilization.

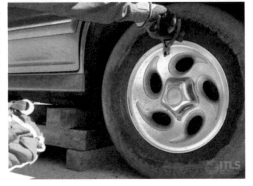

Fig. 43 Pull the tire valve stems after proper cribbing has been completed.

STABILIZATION

Stabilization is a critical aspect of scene safety. Every vehicle is considered unstable upon initial evaluation. The reason vehicles are stabilized in all positions is for the safety and well-being of the rescuers and to prevent further injury to the victim.

As soon as scene safety is assured, the first rescuers on scene should assure that the vehicle ignition is in the "off" position, and the vehicle is in park and/or the parking brake is applied (Fig. 40).

When properly stabilized, the vehicle should have no movement. This task can be accomplished in a relatively short period of time. Thus, there is no excuse to work in, on, or around an unsafe, unstable vehicle. This chapter addresses the stabilization process to assure the safety of everyone.

Car on its wheels

With most motor vehicle collisions, vehicles are found upright and on their wheels. However, never assume that such a vehicle is stable. The first step is to chock the wheels in the position found. This prevents the vehicle from moving once the rescuer gains access. **Never assume the car will not move even when a flat tire is evident.** The next step in the stabilization process is to build box cribs under the frame. The objective is to fill the void and reduce the potential for unpredictable movement.

To build box cribs under the "A" pillars and ahead of the rear wheels (Fig. 41), brace against the wheel well and lift the side of the car, taking the spring action out of the body as another rescuer slides the cribbing in place.

Repeat this procedure for the rear wheel and then the other side (Fig. 42). Always remember to use proper body mechanics with legs for lifting.

With the vehicle braced against the cribbing, take the side cutters from the tool kit and walk around the car pulling the valve stems (Fig. 43). As the suspension system relaxes, it will further tighten the car against the cribbing.

Car on its side

Vehicles on their sides are potentially hazardous to the rescuers and to the victims. Thus, for safety precautions, spotters should be placed at the front and rear of the vehicle to announce any sudden, unpredictable movement. Stabilization of the vehicle on its side consists of filling the contact points between the ground and the vehicle on the undercarriage, and at the roof pillars. Stabilizations devices such as four-by-four hardwood cribbing can accomplish this task. There are other devices on the market that can achieve this objective but are not incorporated in this module. A spare tire gathered at the scene (not from the victim's overturned car) can be utilized as a temporary stabilization device; however, you must assure that the vehicle is resting on the metal wheel and not the tire. When considering stabilization for a vehicle on its side, also simultaneously consider the extrication pathway.

Car on its side — resting on the roof edge

Most cars will balance on the roof edge or drip mold, with the wheels not touching the ground (Fig. 44). This is perhaps the most dangerous position, as the car could roll onto the rescuer or continue onto the roof when touched, thus causing tragic results to those inside the vehicle.

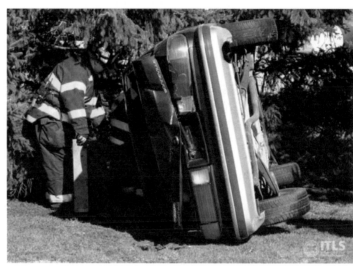

To stabilize a vehicle in this position, plan ahead to determine how to remove the victim(s). The easiest extrication method is to cut the roof on the upper side and lay it down.

Start by building a box crib and sliding it under the rear wheel (Fig. 45).

Fig. 44 Is this car stable?

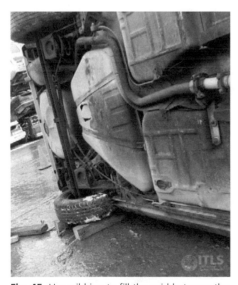

Fig. 45 Use cribbing to fill the void between the wheel and the ground.

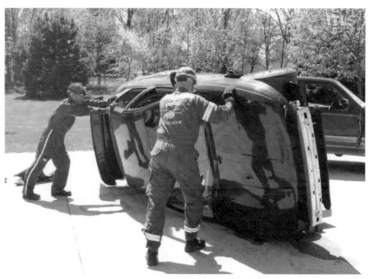

Fig. 46 Bring the vehicle to a 90 degree position for rescuer safety and stabilization.

Position rescuers at opposite ends of the vehicle and gently push the car onto the cribbing (Fig. 46). There is some minimal movement of the vehicle and potential movement of the victims inside. However, the safety of personnel should not be risked by having them enter the vehicle until it is rendered safe.

The cribbing should be centered on the metal wheel rather than the tire (Fig. 47). As one rescuer holds the vehicle in place by pushing on the roof, use the Quik Bar to make a hole in the cowling behind the hood (in front of the windshield), and rotate the Quik Bar to a vertical position, pulling down on it gently. Corrugate the hole and make easy access to the notch-style bumper jack. Place the jack on the ground beneath the hole and insert the blade (Fig. 48-49). Jack only until tight. Do not lift the vehicle.

The Hi-Lift jack or the bumper jack could also be placed into the trunk deck (Fig. 50).

In this case, the cribbing is placed under the front wheel.

Always crib and stabilize on a diagonal. The rescuer should never crib at a 180° position as this causes a pivot point upon which the car could rotate.

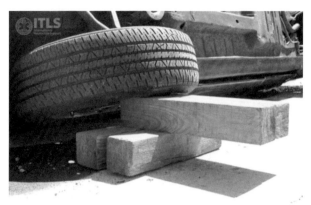

Fig. 47 The cribbing is positioned so the metal rim comes in contact with the cribbing. Photograph is exaggerated to illustrate this point.

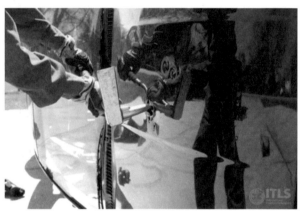

Fig. 48 Using a striking tool, make a purchase point for the stabilization device.

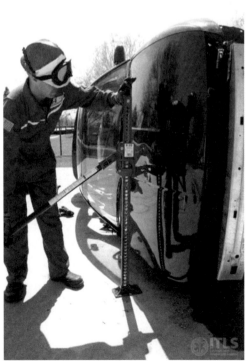

Fig. 49 Make sure the stabilization device is secure.

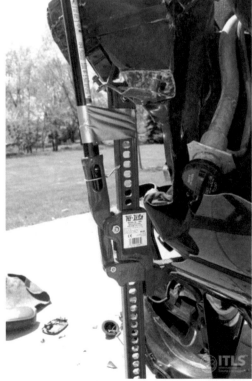

Fig. 50 Make sure the handle has been secured.

Car on its side — resting on tire edge

A car on its side and resting on the tire edge is virtually the same situation as resting on the roof edge, but more stable (Fig. 51). The ideal situation would be to move the vehicle into a 90° position by again placing cribbing under the rear wheel. However, the weight of most cars will preclude this method. Instead, stabilize the vehicle as it is found. The Quik Bar is utilized to make the opening, and the jack is positioned in either the front cowling or trunk deck. Again, it is vitally important not to lift the car.

Car on its roof

Normally, a car on its roof will come to rest with its nose down because of the engine weight. However, some will balance on the roof. This presents stability problems as the vehicle will tend to rotate. If this is the case, place the spare tire under the center of the hood front. (Fig. 52-53).

Next, place some type of cribbing in front of the "A" pillars. This is the void space between the front window frame ("A" pillar) and the ground. The rescuer should then make openings in the "C" pillars (Fig. 54-55).

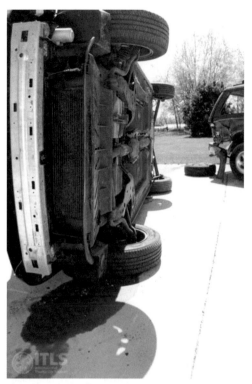

Fig. 51 Vehicles found on the "tire edge" may look secure, but cribbing is still required.

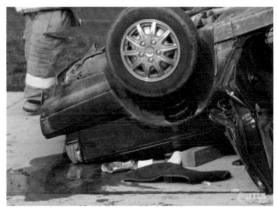

Fig. 52 Cribbing the "A" pillar location will add stability to the vehicle.

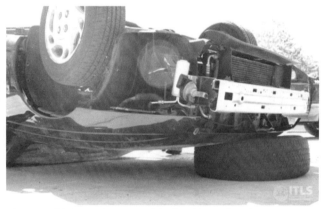

Fig. 53 Cribbing can be accomplished with items found on scene, such as a spare tire.

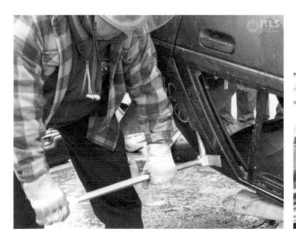

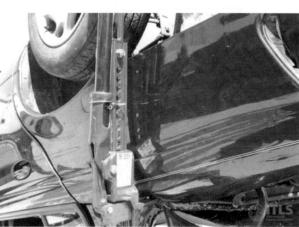

Fig. 54 (left) Make a purchase point for a stabilization device in a vehicle constructed with sheet metal.

Fig. 55 (right) Placement of stabilization devices will differ on vehicles made of composite fiber.

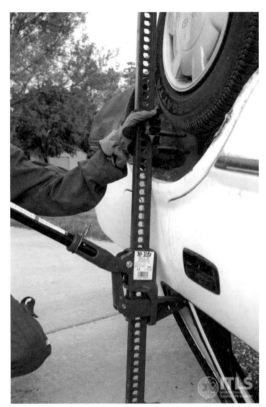

Fig. 56 Utilize areas readily available as points of stability.

Finally, raise the jack until it has made solid contact with the vehicle. If a spare tire was used under the front hood and a void space still exists, raise the car until there is solid contact with the spare tire. REMEMBER: Never lift the vehicle. Only stabilize it.

Vehicles equipped with opera windows or slit glass adapt very well to this method by breaking the glass to insert the jacks (Fig. 56).

Also crib the rear of the roof at the rear window (Fig. 57).

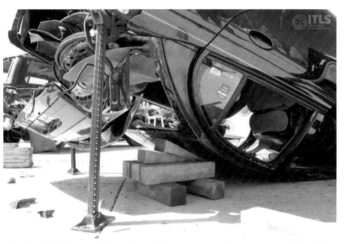

Fig. 57 Cribbing can help with stability or serve as the primary stabilization.

Key Points to Remember

■ Do not puncture tires to flatten.

■ NEVER return car to upright position with victim inside.

■ When using jack, stabilize only. DO NOT LIFT!

■ For safety and to avoid accidental release, secure handle of Hi-Lift jack in upright position.

■ All vehicles involved in a collision are considered to be unstable.

■ Never return a car to its upright position with victims inside.

■ Scene size-up should simultaneously identify and eliminate all hazards.

■ When considering the access point, remember not to interfere with stabilization devices and simultaneously think of the extrication pathway.

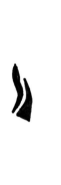

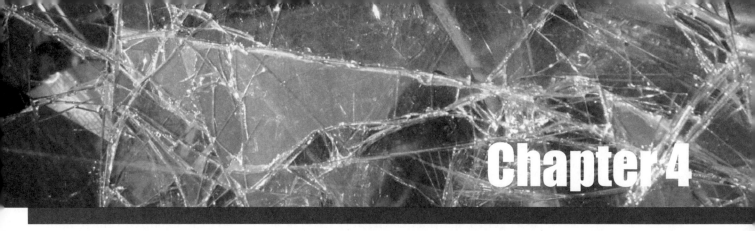

Chapter 4

Accessing

Knowledge Objectives

The rescuer should be able to...

- Determine an access point in a vehicle
- Describe the different types of glass in a vehicle and the tools and the procedures for safely breaking glass
- List the mechanics of securing a door
- Describe the "crash zones" of vehicles
- Describe the sequence of steps in opening doors from either a hinge or bolt mechanism
- Determine when a roof should be removed
- Describe the sequence for removing a roof back to front
- Describe the sequence for dropping a roof from a vehicle on its side
- Describe the sequence for removing the floor assembly from a vehicle
- List the problems and solutions of an engine or trunk compartment fire

Skill Objectives

The rescuer should be able to...

- Safely break tempered and safety glass
- Open a door conventionally
- Expose and cut the "Nader" bolt
- Expose and cut the hinges on doors
- Remove doors
- Unbolt doors
- Remove a roof from back to front
- Drop a roof from a vehicle on its side
- Remove the floor assembly of a vehicle
- Extinguish an engine or trunk compartment fire

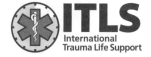

ACCESSING

Remember: Victims should not be accessed until the vehicle is stabilized.

New car construction and design requires all emergency responders to use extra caution when accessing a vehicle with an entrapped victim. The greatest **potential** dangers are any of the supplemental restraint systems (SRS) that can be found anywhere in the passenger compartment. The very first rescuer to enter the stabilized vehicle must take a few seconds to scan the entire interior of the vehicle for SRS. Look specifically for any identification marks or symbols indicating an SRS system located within that portion of the vehicle. The second step is to pass this information onto a partner and other rescuers on scene. Please see Chapter 1 for more details.

Windows

Gaining access into a vehicle through a window can be done quickly and should be regarded as a "starting" place and the last resort route to remove victims for rescue. There are two types of glass in today's automobiles, safety glass and tempered glass.

Safety Glass

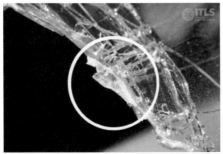
Fig. 58 Safety glass is made with a laminate.

Safety glass is a composition glass molded like a sandwich, consisting of a layer of Butacite® between two layers of glass (Fig. 58). The Butacite® acts as a stiffener and adheres itself to the plate glass as the glass is formed under high heat and pressure.

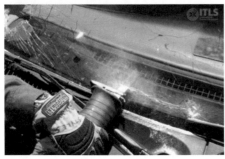
Fig. 59 Glass dust will be a safety concern when laminate glass is cut.

Safety glass will crack very easily but will not come apart due to the lamination between the layers. The design of safety glass will help keep occupants inside of a vehicle and will also work in reverse as a net, preventing objects that may hit the windshield from entering the vehicle. In most cars the windshield is the only glass that is safety glass.

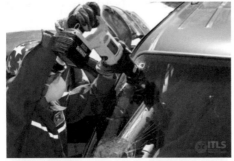
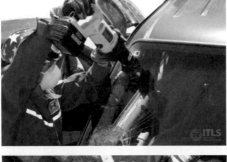
Fig. 60 A reciprocating saw should be used with caution but is considered the preferred tool.

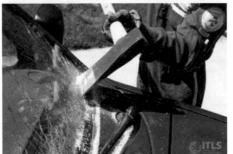
Fig. 61 A striking tool can be used to cut laminate glass.

Safety glass can be removed and pulled off in large shards. Caution must be used by the rescuers to protect themselves and the victims, due to the fine glass powder that the safety glass produces (Fig. 59).

In older model vehicles, a windshield knife could be used to completely remove the glass. In the early 1980s, the vehicle manufacturers changed the mastic used to hold in the glass, thus virtually eliminating the effectiveness of the knife. To remove safety glass windshield in vehicles from the '80s to the present, use a saw (Fig. 60). An axe may be used as a last resort (Fig. 61). Again remembering the amount of glass slivers and dust that safety glass will produce, all safety precautions must be used. Applying shaving cream along the course of the cut in the safety glass will help trap glass dust and small shards.

The windshields of many models of pickup truck and larger truck are set in a rubber molding. Most of these trucks' windshields can be removed by prying up one end of the windshield with a pry tool. Grasping onto the rubber molding with a gloved hand, remove the rubber, which will remove the windshield.

Tempered Glass

All remaining glass in automobiles will be tempered glass. This glass is also formed under high heat and pressure into a tough sheet without lamination. Tempered glass has a memory (Fig. 62). It will bend without cracking. In most collisions, tempered glass may be hit with a blunt object without breaking. A sharp object, such as a spring-loaded center punch or a point of an axe, will shatter tempered glass very easily, into thousands of quarter-inch shards. These shards, although they do not look dangerous, are very sharp. Tempered glass will not normally produce the powder associated with safety glass.

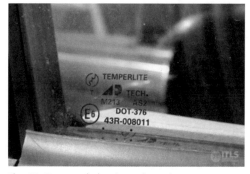

Fig. 62 Tempered glass is made to shatter.

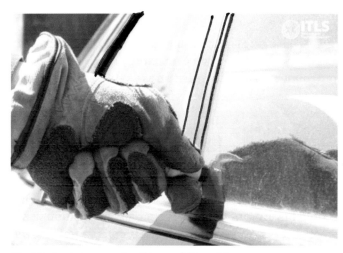

Fig. 63 A window punch will be useful in gaining access.

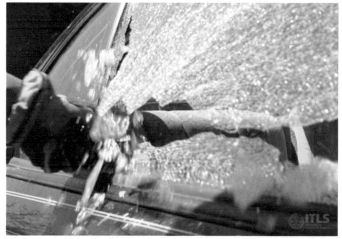

Fig. 64 Proper PPEs should be used when attempting a window punch.

The best means of access through tempered glass is the use of a spring-loaded center punch placed in a lower corner of the window located the furthest away from any victims (Fig. 63-64).

Many vehicles today have laminated sun tinting on the inside of the window, which will prevent the thousands of pieces of glass from falling into the vehicle or on the victim. If time will allow, you should consider the use of duct tape or contact paper over the window, which will hold the glass together after it has shattered, again not allowing the thousands of pieces of broken glass to fall on the victim. This is particularly important if the vehicle is on its side or on the roof. Push gently on any corner of the window with the center punch; following through will shatter the glass. A few shards may still remain and may need to be brushed away (Fig. 65).

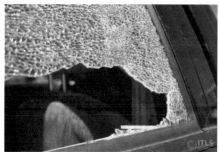

Fig. 65 Tempered glass is designed to break into small shards, but the glass will still cut.

If a spring-loaded center punch is not available, other sharp pointed objects may be used to shatter the glass. A long, flat blade screwdriver (Fig. 66), the flat blade end of a lug wrench, a car aerial, and an engine dip stick can all be used in a whipping action.

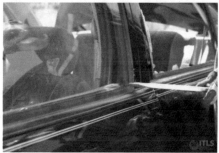

Fig. 66 Other tools can be used to shatter tempered glass.

If glass does not shatter with whatever tool you are using to strike the tempered glass, consider that some newer vehicles are

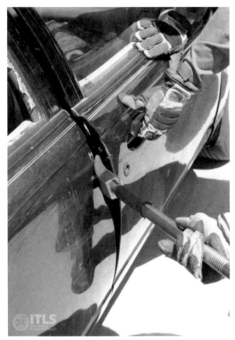

Fig. 67 Remember to "try before you pry."

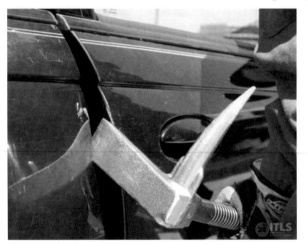

Fig. 68 When making an attempt to force a door open, consider the vehicle's body type (sheet metal vs. composite fiber).

constructed with laminated (or other types of safety glass) around the entire vehicle. Cutting as discussed previously may be your best option.

When shattering glass, always work away from the victim if possible. Also, clean away as much of the glass as possible before proceeding. **ALWAYS** remember your personal protective equipment (PPE), especially your gloves, when removing glass.

Doors

When attempting to open or remove a door, it is always important to remember to *try before you pry* (Fig. 67). Don't forget to try the inside and outside latch, at the same time remembering to unlock the door before attempting to open. The mechanics of the door are closing, latching and locking.

Vehicles today have "crash zones" that cause the vehicles to fold at predetermined points. Most doors will open even after a head-on collision. "T-Bone" collisions and rollovers cause doors to jam as well as other problems with getting them open.

The first step is to unlock the door. This can be accomplished by working the manual lock (up, on the mushroom head, or in direction shown on slide locks).

The second step is to determine if the door is jammed. One rescuer should have a door handle in an unlatched position while another rescuer uses the hooligan tool or pinch bar to force the door past the jam (Fig. 68).

If the door opens in this manner, it should be pushed past the normal opening to gain room for extrication. This must be done in a smooth manner so as not to bounce the car around, and only after someone has secured the victim manually for spinal motion restriction.

The latch/lock box is a sophisticated assembly. The scissors of the latch (Fig. 69) will jam around the lock pin ("Nader" bolt) (Fig. 70-71). The pin will not be able to be broken with hand tools.

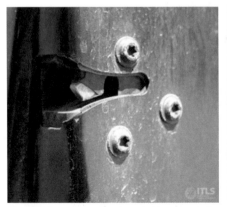

Fig. 69 The "scissor latch" used to secure the doors.

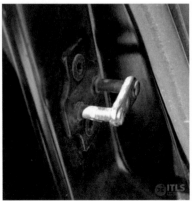

Fig. 70 A common dual lock pin.

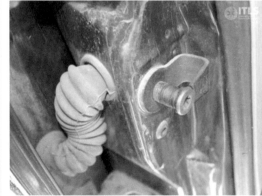

Fig. 71 A common "Nader" bolt.

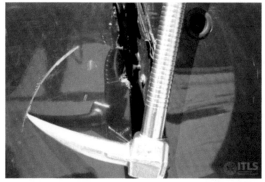

Fig. 72 Creating a purchase point to access the locking or "Nader" pin.

Two methods can be used. With the hooligan tool, bend the lip of the door back to expose the lock bolt (Fig. 72).

Using the reciprocating saw with a small blade, cut through the "Nader" pin (Fig. 73-74). Apply soapy water liberally. The bolt should part in 20 to 30 seconds. Use the hooligan tool to force the door past the jam.

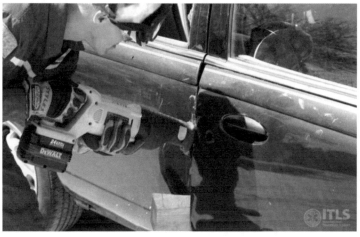

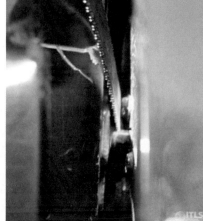

Fig. 73 (left) Cutting the lock or "Nader" pin can be accomplished with a properly placed reciprocating saw.

Fig. 74 (right) Using the right type of reciprocating saw blade will make this task easier.

The second method is to remove the door from the hinge side. There are two types of hinges: cast and formed or stamped. The cast hinge is the tougher of the two (Fig. 75).

The formed or stamped hinge is made of mild steel and is very easy to cut (Fig. 76-77).

The removal techniques are the same. First, you will need to make an opening with the hooligan tool to expose the hinges.

Some vehicles may require the use of the panel cutter to accomplish this (Fig. 78). Other cutting tools (one is similar to a large manual can opener found on a rescue tool) will also create an opening to access the hinges. The reciprocating saw, with a short blade, will also work here.

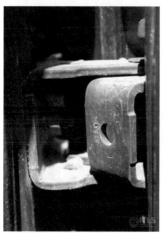

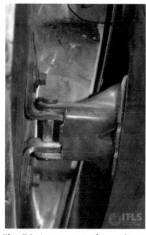

Fig. 75 A common cast type of hinge.

Fig. 76 A common "formed" or "stamped" type of hinge.

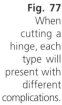

Fig. 77 When cutting a hinge, each type will present with different complications.

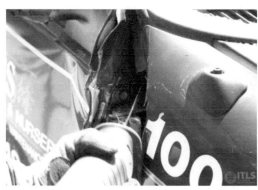

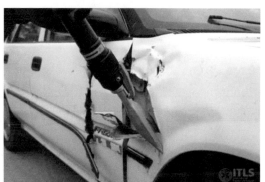

Fig. 78 Cutting the sheet-metal body of the vehicle will allow more room for accessing the hinges.

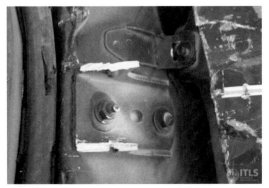

Fig. 79 Cutting through the hinges will allow the removal of a door, giving the rescuer access to the victim.

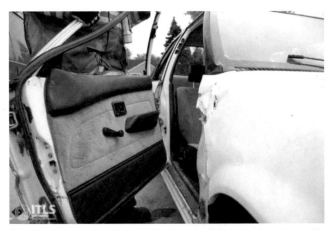

Fig. 80 After cutting through the hinges, pulling the door back will allow for more access room.

Once exposed, cut the hinges with the reciprocating saw (Fig. 79). The size of the blade will be determined after you expose the hinges. In most cases, the short blade is used so as not to "bottom out." This can be prevented by placing the blade on the edge closest to you and then moving the blade in across the hinge. If you proceed too fast, the blade will strike the other side. When cutting a lock bolt (or "Nader" pin), this technique may also prevent a "bottoming out."

Once the hinges are cut, bend the door back on the lock in a circular motion (Fig. 80).

In most instances, the "Nader" pin will pull loose from the scissors. Caution must be used, and it is important to have someone holding the door in case the scissors let go unexpectedly, because the door can possibly injure your feet. After the door is removed, it is important to have someone carry the door far enough away, where it will not be in the way of the rest of your rescue.

Removing the door, whether it is front or rear, is done in the same manner. The latch/lock systems are virtually the same.

An additional method for removing the rear door is by unbolting it. When the front door is removed on most cars, it reveals the hinges on the rear door (Fig. 81).

There are typically three bolts. These bolts can usually be removed with a 1/2" or 9/16" socket; if they are metric, the sizes should be 14 or 15 mm. At times, this can be accomplished with open end or box wrenches. Many new vehicles will have the hinges attached without the use of any bolts, or a combination of a bolt, or a 'rivet' type of bolt. If this is seen, then proceed to cut the hinges, as unbolting them will not be an option.

Chapter Six on Disentanglement will discuss removing the entire side or dropping the side.

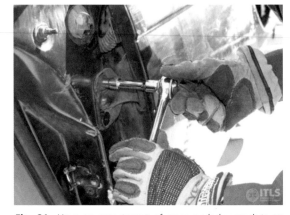

Fig. 81 Have an assortment of open-ended wrenches or sockets to unbolt the door hinges.

Roofs

In some instances, a roof may need to be removed to gain access and remove victims. This should only be done when the safety and quick extrication of the victim makes it necessary. Roofs should not be removed just for the sake of removing them. Cost of the vehicle should not be a factor when deciding whether to remove a roof. When possible, rescuers can gain access through a door or a window to protect the victim prior to and during the roof removal.

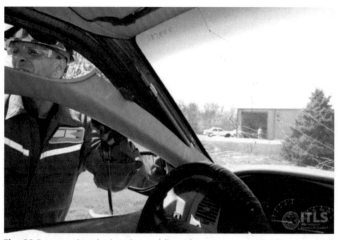

Fig. 82 By removing the interior molding, the rescuer can visualize potential hazards while speeding up the cutting process.

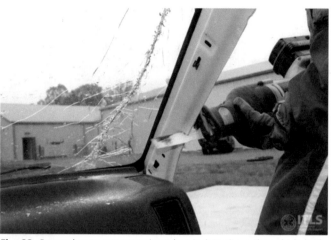

Fig. 83 Remember to cut approximately 4 inches above the vehicle body and away from the patient.

Some of the factors that would warrant taking the time to remove the roof are: severe entrapment, type of victim injuries, location of vehicle (ditches), and the fastest way out for the victim.

The removal procedure is very simple with either a hand-held hacksaw or a reciprocating saw. Prior to the first cuts, make sure a rescuer has completed the scan of the passenger compartment for any Supplemental Restraint Systems. These restraint system locations will be marked or labeled (look along the "A," "B," and "C" pillars and inside roof molding). Remove any plastic or molding. Rescuers can now see the exact SRS locations, and avoid cutting into them. Much time can also be saved if the doors are opened first. This will avoid the need to cut the window frames. Start with the "A" pillar and cut at right angles about four inches up from the dash (Fig. 82-83).

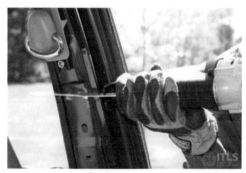

Fig. 84 Consider potential hazards and structural reinforcements found in the "B" pillar.

Cut all the way through the windshield. Next, cut the "B" pillars within two inches of the top (Fig. 84). Then the "C" pillars. If you are using a hand hacksaw, it is important to look and see the shortest distance glass to glass (door opening to the rear window) (Fig. 85).

Start the cut from the front to the rear on an angle (never straight). The "C" pillar may be too wide for the saw frame. If it is, cut a pie-shaped wedge from the rear and finish off the cut. Take advantage of opera windows in this phase of the cut.

When using the reciprocating saw, use up and down strokes. Let the saw do the work while keeping a steady pressure, and the guard (boot: flat part) flush and in complete contact with the material being cut. This will prevent the blade from bending during your cut. Another rescuer should keep a good spray

Fig. 85 Cutting any post can also be accomplished with a hacksaw.

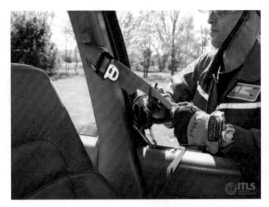

Fig. 86 (above) Remember to cut the seat belts prior to roof removal. Cut in a diagonal direction.

Fig. 87 (right) Roof flap can be performed with two rescuers. Remember that glass should never go over the victim.

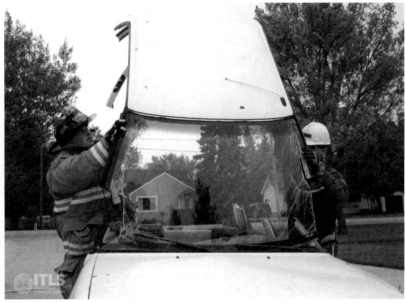

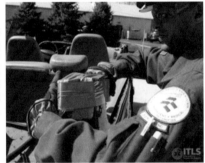

Fig. 88 Safety first: Cover exposed sharp edges to prevent injury.

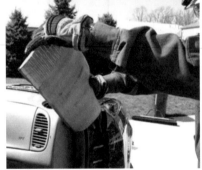

Fig. 89 Old or non-compliant hose lengths can be put to use covering sharp edges.

from the soap bottle on the saw blade. To ensure quick cutting, a new blade and solid pressure of the swivel foot to the surface to be cut should be used.

When all the pillars are severed, cut the seat belts (Fig. 86) and, with another rescuer on the far side, lift the roof to a vertical position from the rear to the front (Fig. 87). The windshield will tear away at the base, and the roof will be placed upside down on the hood. By using this method, glass will not pass over the victim(s). Be sure to cover any exposed pillar ends with duct tape (Fig. 88-89).

If the vehicle is upright, in most incidences cutting a flap in a roof takes just as much time. If the roof is removed as described above, access to the victim will be the best it can be.

Airway management, patient assessment, placement of cervical collars, and treatment in general are tremendously enhanced when there is room to move around and to see clearly.

Dropping the Roof of a Car Lying on Its Side

Slide a full spine board into the rear window to protect the victim(s) (Fig. 90). Cut the uppermost "A" (Fig. 91), "B" (if there is one) (Fig. 92), and "C" pillars (Fig. 93) as directed for the car on its wheels. Remember to locate any SRS located along the roof rail.

When cutting the "A" pillars, allow the saw to cut the bottom of the windshield all

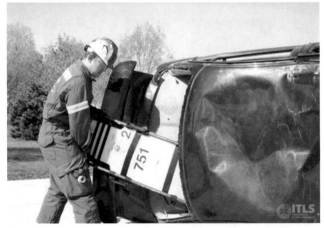

Fig. 90 Remember to protect the victim before cutting or prying.

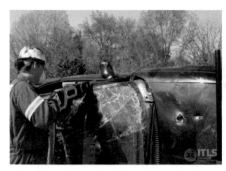

Fig. 91 Remember to cut at least 4 inches above the body of the vehicle.

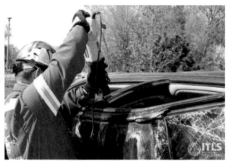

Fig. 92 Don't forget to clear the molding before cutting the post.

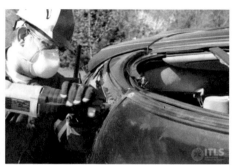

Fig. 93 Consider potential hazards found in the "C" pillar.

the way to the lower "A" pillar (Fig. 94-95). Cut this pillar half-way through (Fig. 96). Remove any tempered glass that is in the way in both the side or rear windows.

Reach in and cut the "B" pillar (if there is one) halfway through and repeat on the "C" pillar.

All these "halfway" cuts are from the inside down toward the outside, so that it is possible to bend the entire roof downward (Fig. 97) (after having cut the upper seat belt).

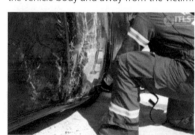

Fig. 94 While cutting down safety glass, remember the potential glass dust and dash.

This will ensure the stability of the car as the roof will not be entirely removed (Fig. 98).

Cover all sharp edges of the severed pillars with duct tape, hose sections, multi-trauma dressings, or other such material that may be available. (Fig. 99-100).

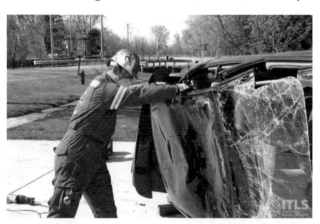

Fig. 95 Cut approximately 4 inches above the vehicle body and away from the victim.

There may be times that this procedure may not be possible. It may be better to use the reciprocal saw to cut only the tin of the roof; one across the top, around 12" from the edge, two down cuts, one in the front, one in the rear, again 10 to 12 inches from the edge. Flap the roof down

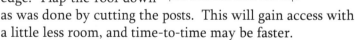

Fig. 96 Cutting half-way through the "A" pillar allows an easier roof flap.

as was done by cutting the posts. This will gain access with a little less room, and time-to-time may be faster.

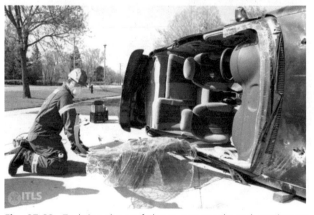

Fig. 97-98 To bring the roof down, use gentle and continuous pressure. Remember to communicate with the victim during access.

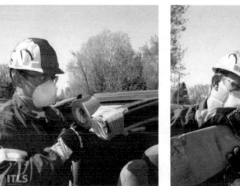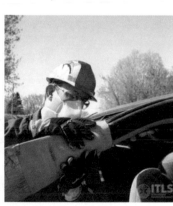

Fig. 99-100 An ounce of prevention will go a long way.

Fig. 101
Floor drains
are a good
initial
purchase
point.

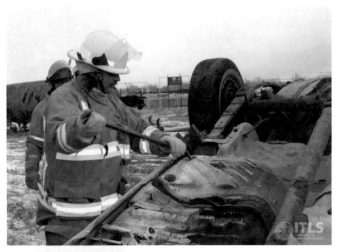

Floors

The floor assembly in most vehicles is the least reinforced and most easily breached part of the vehicle. The vehicle may come to rest on its side into a building, upside down in a ditch, or in some other position that requires access to the passenger compartment through the bottom of the vehicle, as the doors or roof are inaccessible. Use caution; the catalytic converter may be hot and can cause injury.

The first step is to clean off the bottom of the vehicle. Use the power saw to cut the drive shaft at the universal joint and pull it down toward the rear to slide it out of the spline in the transmission and discard it. Next, cut the brake cables and cut off the exhaust system. All gas lines must be cut and plugged before stripping the vehicle bottom. See section on hybrid vehicles in Chapter 1 for identification of power cables.

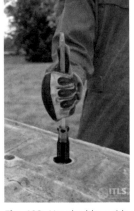

Fig. 102 Use the blunt side to prevent victim injury.

The foot well in the rear seat is obvious when viewed from the bottom. Punch out the drain hole covers, providing an opening for the reciprocating saw (Fig. 101).

A short saw blade should be used to avoid hitting the victim or objects in the vehicle such as the seat. Push the handle of the large screwdriver through the hole to make sure no body parts are near the intended saw path (Fig. 102).

Cut the metal or composite then push the rug away. This will help eliminate the problem of potentially cutting the occupants. Make a three-sided cut the full size of the raised portion of the floor pan (Fig. 103).

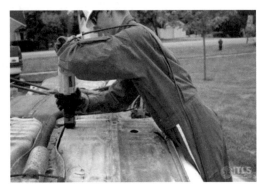

Fig. 103 Making the initial entry point for rescuers.

Bend back the flap and push the rug in and out of the way (Fig. 104). At this time, with the hole in the floor, you should be able to determine if any of the victims are in the way.

One or two rescuers can now enter through the opening to stabilize the victim(s), (Fig. 105). Use duct tape around the sharp edges of the opening before entering.

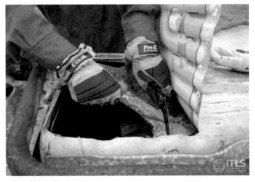

Fig. 104 By making a three-cut flap, a rescuer can gain entry to evaluate the victims.

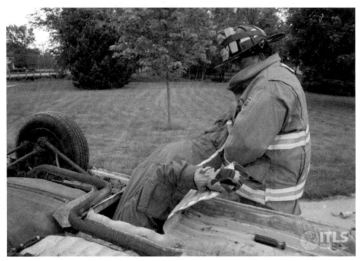

Fig. 105 By allowing a rescuer access into the vehicle, triage can begin.

When removing the entire floor, run the reciprocating saw around the perimeter of the passenger compartment. The only problems normally encountered are around the transmission therefore it may be necessary to cut the support brackets.

Next, cut the seat belts to the front seat. With the long pinch bar and hooligan tool, pry the entire floor out from the car along with the front seat attached. The entire passenger compartment will be exposed.

Engine Compartment

Firewalls on most vehicles have large holes in them to accommodate heater/air-conditioning components, and these holes and the heater/air-conditioning components are usually made of plastic (Fig. 106-107).

The transfer of heat, smoke and fire can occur very rapidly from the engine compartment into the passenger area. It is imperative that a fire be stopped in its incipient stage when persons are trapped.

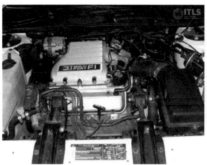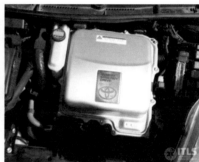
Fig. 106-107 Different vehicle types bring different engine compartment issues.

Immediately upon arrival, if there is smoke around the engine compartment, try to release the hood by holding and pulling the hood latch. Have another rescuer stand by with an ABC extinguisher. If flames are visible, do not do this without full protective gear in place.

Do not waste time trying to force the hood. Using the pike end of the hooligan tool, drive it through the hood in at least four places, one foot on either side of the center (Fig. 108). Do not penetrate the middle of the hood. This will avoid hitting the air cleaner.

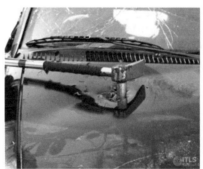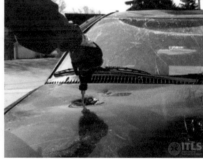
Fig. 108 Making the hole in the hood is the first step in fire containment. **Fig. 109** Push the hood insulation out of the way before discharging the extinguisher.

Next, push the long screwdriver through the holes to free them of insulation (Fig. 109).

Hold the extinguisher nozzle in the holes and discharge it in short bursts (Fig. 110).

If a garden hose is available nearby, use it!

The threat of fire is the one event in which all other actions are put aside to concentrate on victim removal. While one rescuer tries to contain the fire, the other works on the victim(s). The above fire suppression technique should only be attempted if there are victims remaining in the vehicles and fire

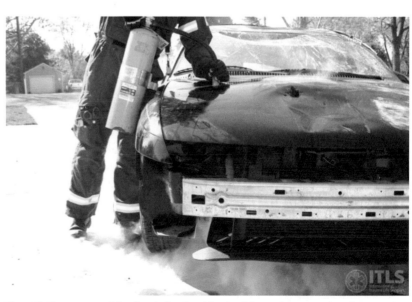
Fig. 110 Short spurts of dry chemical extinguisher in all four points can reduce fire spread.

service is not on scene. If there are no victims in the vehicle, allow fire department personnel to extinguish the fire when they arrive.

Trunk Compartment

The trunk can be especially hazardous because people tend to use it as a storage locker.

Flammable materials (such as books, papers, cartons, clothing, and gasoline) and explosive materials (such as spare tires, air cans, aerosol cans and many others too numerous to mention) can create a HAZMAT condition. The transfer of a fire into the passenger compartment would be quicker than from the front end, as it is usually wide open behind the rear seat cushion.

In case there is a fire, do not open the trunk due to the risk of a HAZMAT explosion. Instead, using the pinch bar or hooligan tool, smash out the rear lights — they usually extend into the trunk compartment. Next, spray an extinguishing agent through the opening.

Once again, while one rescuer is taking care of this task, the other is working to free and remove the victim(s).

Never leave the scene of any collision without first checking all vehicle trunks of the cars involved. It is entirely possible that persons could be in the trunk at the time of the collision and be knocked unconscious. College hazing is just one example of when a victim could be locked in the trunk.

Key Points to Remember

- Note the placement of the center punch at the lower corner of the window. This restricts "follow through" of the hand.

- When using a striking tool to break glass, the motion should be with the wrist.

- All glass will cut when broken.

- Doors are the preferred mode of entry and egress.

- If doors are jammed on one side, try the other side before starting forcible entry.

- No amount of force on a pry bar will break the door latch!

- When cutting anything, lubricate liberally with soapy water.

- Use a generic dishwashing detergent mixed with water 6 parts to 1. Put the water in the spray bottle first and add the detergent to prevent suds.

- Use a small (4") saw blade if the problem of "bottoming out" is a possibility.

- Cast hinges are harder to cut than stamped or pressed hinges. Be careful that the door does not drop if a cast hinge shatters.

- Roof removal gives much more room to provide victim care, protect the cervical spine and secure the airway.

- Flapping the roof requires more effort and time than removing it altogether.

- It is usually not necessary to cut the bottom of the windshield when removing the roof from rear to front. The windshield will tear away. This will also reduce the risk of glass falling on the victim.

- If gas lines are metal, crimp them with pliers before cutting.

- Be aware that catalytic converters can be extremely hot.

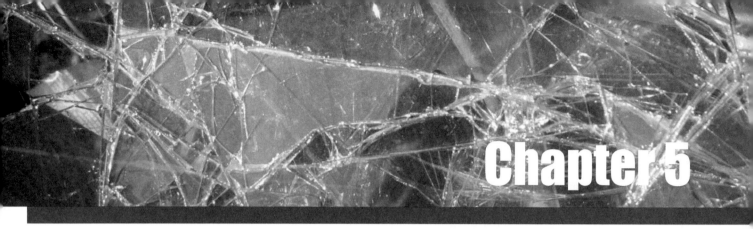

Chapter 5

Stabilizing the Victim

Knowledge Objectives

The rescuer should be able to...

- Summarize the sequence of the assessment and the stabilization of the trauma victim

- Describe the steps of the in-vehicle emergency care procedures

- Describe steps that can be used to protect the victim from further injury

Skill Objectives

The rescuer should be able to...

- Carry out the assessment and emergency care of the trauma victims

- Protect the victim from further injury

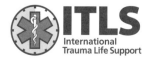

ITLS
International
Trauma Life Support

STABILIZING THE VICTIM

Assessment and Immediate Care

Gaining safe access to the victim allows the rescuers to apply their knowledge and skills gained from their trauma education. In addition to patient care, rescuers must also be planning how they will package and remove (extricate) the victim.

Access courses allow students to practice both their skills as trauma care providers and rescuers in a controlled but realistic environment. A detailed discussion of the assessment and management of the multiple trauma victim is beyond the scope of this course. This chapter serves only as a reminder of the key points of trauma assessment and care for the entrapped victim due to a motor vehicle collision. It does not replace a complete ITLS course.

Too many times EMS units are not taught under realistic conditions. How many have been taught how to apply a cervical collar while sitting upright in a kitchen chair? This is totally unrealistic. Try practicing on real people in various pretzel-like positions in wrecked cars. There is quite a difference! Rescuers should be trained and practice using the most realistic methods possible.

Assessment of the victim(s) should follow the steps outlined in the ITLS primary and secondary survey. The ITLS primary survey is designed to identify those problems that pose an immediate threat to the victim's life.

Assessment of the victim in a motor vehicle collision really begins during the dispatch of the call, when clues to the mechanism of injury are given during the report. Upon arrival, assess the scene for safety, mitigate hazards, determine the number of victims and mobilize the necessary resources.

Begin with the initial assessment. Assess the airway for patency while protecting the cervical spine. If it is not patent, open the airway using the chin-lift, jaw-thrust method. Any obstructions, such as blood, vomitus or foreign bodies, must be cleared, using suction or the obstructed airway maneuver. All trauma victims should receive supplemental high flow oxygen.

Breathing is assessed for rate and adequacy. If the breathing is inadequate, assist the victim's respiration with a pocket mask or bag-valve mask (BVM). If the victim is unable to protect their airway (absent gag) or there is a significant risk of losing the airway, secure the airway using endotracheal intubation, a blind insertion airway device (BIAD) or other airway adjunct, depending on level of training.

Listen to the chest for presence of breath sounds. Absent breath sounds and tracheal deviation away from the injured side are signs of a tension pneumothorax. This should be relieved by needle decompression, as soon as possible.

Assess the circulation by checking for presence of both a carotid and radial pulse. Absence of a radial pulse with carotid pulses present indicates that the victim may be going into shock. Also remember that a rapid pulse in the presence of good perfusion may represent the earliest sign of shock. IV access and fluid resuscitation should not be attempted in the vehicle unless you are faced with a prolonged extrication problem. In critical victims, IVs should be started en route to the hospital.

Assess the neurological status of the victim to stimuli, using the AVPU method. Altered levels of consciousness may be due to head trauma, poor perfusion or hypoxia. Do not assume that the victim is unconscious "because they are drunk."

The initial assessment should take less than 90 seconds, in most cases. It should be interrupted only to correct potentially life-threatening conditions that have been identified in the primary survey. Remember that any victim with a problem identified in the primary survey should be classified as a "Load and Go," requiring rapid extrication and prompt transport. Given the mechanism of injury, it is rare that these victims would be considered to have the cervical spine cleared in the field setting and should all receive spinal motion restriction.

This is only a brief overview of assessment and intervention. For a more complete explanation of the process, reference the ITLS textbook. Remember also that while assessment and care have begun during this phase of the rescue, they must be continued throughout the rest of the rescue and during transport to the hospital.

Protecting the Victim

Many times, little thought is given to protecting the victim from further injury. Once inside the vehicle and the primary survey is started, determine what extra measures must be taken to protect the head, eyes, ears, etc. Make sure the victim(s) are shielded from glass fragments. Use a blanket, tarpaulin, turn-out coat or even a newspaper found in the vehicle (Fig. 111).

Environmental conditions such as heat or cold can adversely affect trauma victims (and rescue personnel). Be aware of the potential for problems such as hypothermia, inhalation of exhaust fumes from rescue vehicles and tools, and dehydration and/or exhaustion in your personnel.

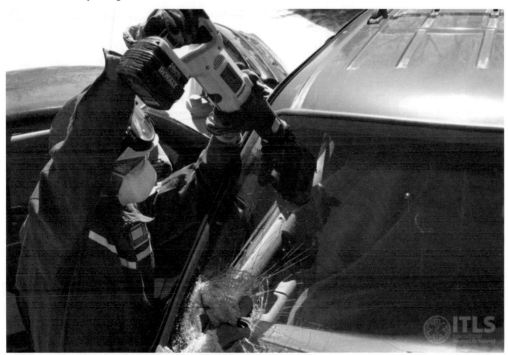

Fig. 111 Remember to protect the victim while gaining access.

Key Points to Remember

- Primary Survey (Fig. 112):
    - o "A" - Airway with C-spine protection
    - o "B" - Breathing assessment and support
    - o "C" - Circulatory assessment and support
    - o "D" – Disability- rapid, brief mental status assessment
    - o "E" – Expose / Environment

    Any problem identified in the primary survey means that the victim meets "Load and Go" criteria.

- Do not delay transport except to manage the airway. If the airway cannot be secured quickly, use an alternative method and repeat attempts for the definitive airway en route. IVs should be established en route to the hospital, unless there is going to be a prolonged extrication.

- Absence of radial pulses suggests shock.

- Mental status exam:
    - o "A" - Victim is ALERT
    - o "V" - Victim responds to VERBAL stimuli
    - o "P" - Victim responds to PAIN
    - o "U" -Victim is UNRESPONSIVE

- Victims who are drunk do die! Those under the influence of any intoxicant may not present in the expected manner. Failure to be aware of this may lead to a preventable death.

- Care of the victim is an on-going process.

- Perform the ITLS ongoing assessment frequently.

- Provide psychological support:
    - o Talk to the victim.
    - o Provide information about what is happening.

- Watch for environmental stresses (hypothermia/hyperthermia) in victims and personnel.

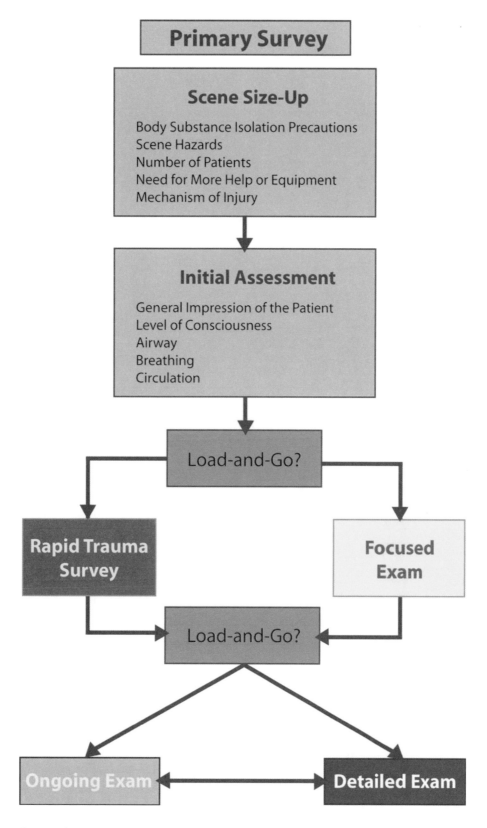

Fig. 112 The ITLS Primary Assessment.

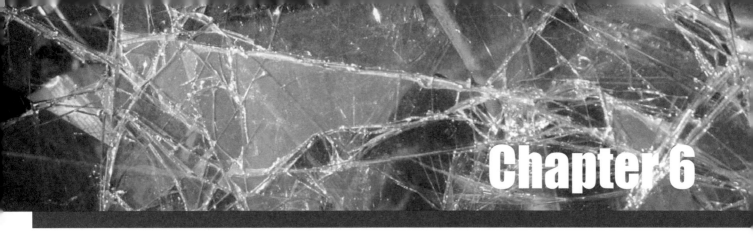

Disentanglement

Knowledge Objectives

The rescuer should be able to...

- Summarize the disentanglement phase of vehicle rescue
- Describe removing the battery cable
- Describe methods of removal from steering column/wheel entrapment
- Describe "blowing out" the front end of the vehicle
- Describe disentangling a trapped foot
- Describe dropping the sides of a wrecked vehicle
- Describe lifting a vehicle off a trapped victim

Skill Objectives

The rescuer should be able to...

- Remove the correct battery cable
- Correctly move back a seat
- Remove the steering wheel rim and column
- "Blow out" the front end
- Disentangle a trapped foot
- Drop the sides of a wrecked vehicle
- Lift a vehicle off a victim trapped underneath

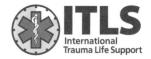

DISENTANGLEMENT

In the case of Access, disentanglement is literally freeing the victim from the wreckage, using only the tools immediately available. This process is likened to peeling an orange. It is very seldom that the victim is impaled; rather, the entrapment results from the wreckage being wrapped around the victim.

Disentanglement is the prelude to packaging. It is accomplished by moving metal or plastic to allow the easy removal of the victim.

Removal of the roof and doors to gain access has been discussed. Now, let's discuss techniques that will quicken the "freeing" process.

In many of today's vehicles, the battery is no longer located in the engine compartment. Rescuers are faced with vehicles that have too many functions that rely on electric power, to have a standard operating procedure which calls for disconnecting power indiscriminately. Attempting to move an electric seat manually quickly reminds the rescuers of the need to be sure of their actions prior to doing anything.

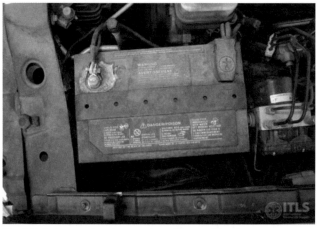

Fig. 113 Before cutting the negative cable, consider the consequences.

Do not cut the battery cables. Remove the negative cable (black) when experiencing an electrical problem (Fig. 113), or to cancel the air bags if they were not deployed. In the absence of an obvious battery, there will usually be one or two posts that appear the same as battery posts. These are designed to allow the disconnection of power to the vehicle. Rescuers can disconnect these as they would a regular battery. CAUTION: Many of the vehicles on the road today have more than one battery. Never take battery disconnection as "fail safe." If there are no apparent problems, do not touch the battery!

Steering Column / Wheel

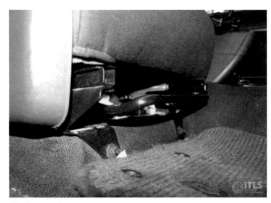

Fig. 114 Moving a seat may give the rescuers more room to access the victim.

Probably the most common cause of entrapment is the steering column/wheel. The old "rig from the frame and pull it out like a bad tooth with a tool on the hood" routine is just that — OLD. Never say never, but there are many more sophisticated ways to solve the problem.

First, try the seat. If it is a mechanical seat, it may have slipped the ratchet and moved forward during the crash. Have another rescuer grasp the seat with both hands (one on front of the seat and one on the top of the back). Trip the seat adjustment lever (remember, the seat is sprung to move forward) (Fig. 114), and gently push the seat back.

A jerky motion, which can be accentuated by the spring action, could seriously jeopardize a C-spine injury.

Do not attempt to move the seat back by yourself.

If the seat is electrically operated, find the right button to move it back (Fig. 115). In addition, especially in luxury cars, locate buttons that power-tilt the steering wheel or a power telescoping column control. These could also provide a little more room.

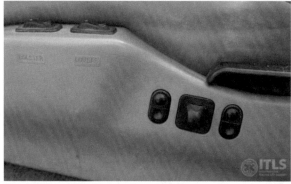
Fig. 115 By cutting the negative cable, the rescuer loses the ability to adjust the electric seats.

Read the directional labels so as not to aggravate the situation by pushing the wrong button. Never attempt to dislodge the seat with mechanical force (hydraulic tools) with the victim in the seat.

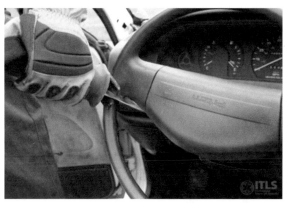
Fig. 116 A hand or power saw can be used effectively to cut the steering wheel.

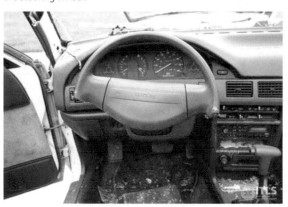
Fig. 117 Cutting the steering wheel may give the rescuer precious inches for gaining access or extricating the victim.

Six to eight inches can be gained by moving a seat back. If unsuccessful, the next step is to remove the steering wheel.

The rim of a steering wheel can be cut easily with either the hand or power saws (Fig. 116). The metal used on the rim is soft steel with no spring action.

Either cut the spokes or bend them out of the way. This action will gain an additional six inches (Fig. 117).

If the car is equipped with an undeployed air bag, disconnect the battery terminals and work around the bag module. Do not cut into the module; it will serve no purpose.

Still not enough room? Remove the steering column not by pulling but by cutting! Though the columns on some cars look awesome because

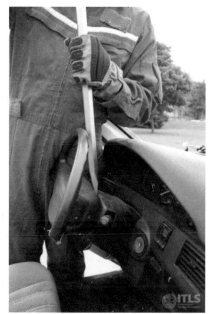

of their size, you must realize the actual steering column is nothing more than a 5/8" or 3/4" mild steel shaft easily cut with the hand saw or power saw once it is stripped.

Use the cold chisel and machinist hammer to peel off the cosmetic plastic covers (Fig. 118).

Fig. 118 Any striking tool and hammer can clear the cosmetic plastic around the steering shaft.

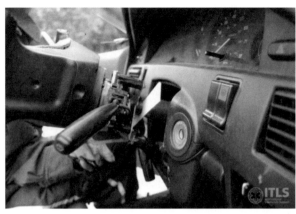 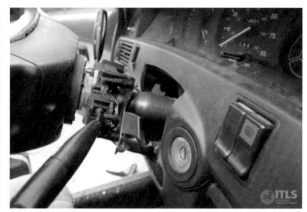

Fig. 119-120 The steering shft is now accessible to the rescuer for cutting.

Note the wiring harness runs down the column (Fig. 119-120). Again, this is a reason to disconnect the battery cable to avoid any sparking when cutting through the column. Having removed the plastic and material surrounding the steering column, the best action is to gently move the wiring harness from the path of any further cuts. This also prevents the remote possibility of hot-starting the car.

Two things to consider: Be sure the victim is protected before cutting commences. Placing a short back board across the legs will suffice. As an added safety, pull the saw upward (this may not be possible, thus the board). Have another rescuer hold the wheel/column so it does not drop when the cut is through.

Be sure to use liberal amounts of soapy water on the saw blade.

Moving the Dash / Front End

There may come a time when the dash is crushed over, preventing all of the previously discussed methods. The answer here is to "blow" the front end out of the car. To even consider a "dash roll" is a waste of time.

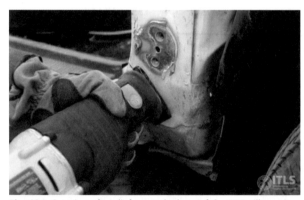

Fig. 121 Creation of a relief cut at the base of the "A" pillar, using a reciprocating saw.

Blowing the front end is a simple maneuver. To begin, the roof has been removed and the doors are open or removed as well.

Next, using the power saw with the long blade, cut on an angle at the base of the "A" pillars toward the front of the vehicle (Fig. 121).

Cut as deep as possible. On a framed auto, only cut the body work. Do not attempt to cut the frame.

Place the Hi-Lift jack with its base against the bottom of the "B" pillar and the lifting lip near the top hinge on the "A" pillar (Fig. 122). Remember

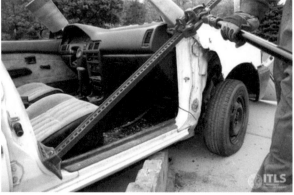

Fig. 122 Proper placement of the Hi-Lift jack for moving the dash.

to place cribbing underneath the "B" pillar; this will prevent a loss of lift or movement through the rocker panel (base of car).

If available, a bumper jack can be placed in a similar position on the opposite side.

Use the Hi-Lift on the side where the victim is located so as to get maximum push (Fig. 123).

Raise the dash by working both jacks simultaneously.

The metal at the bottom "A" post cuts should start tearing almost immediately.

Keep checking the lower extremities of the victim to make sure they do not hang up on the column or pedals.

Raise the dash and crib under the "A" pillars (Fig. 124). Only go as far as needed to free the victim.

Remember, a cardinal rule of rescue: "If an inch is needed, do not go two inches or the victim and rescuers become subjected to possible injury."

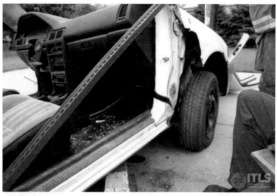

Fig. 123 Actual displacement of the front end. Note the angle of the dash and the front hood.

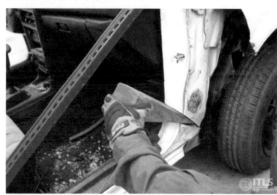

Fig. 124 Use of a piece of wedge cribbing in the relief cut to maintain the position of the front end.

Foot / Floorboard Entrapment

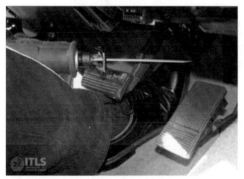

Fig. 125 Position of the reciprocating saw to cut the top of a pedal. Note: Use protection if at all possible. (Protection absent to show position of saw.)

It is common to find a foot encased when the metal floor section folds up under the dash. If the shoe cannot be loosened and the foot slipped out, use the reciprocating saw to cut around the foot and remove the floorboard and victim (Fig. 125). Keep well away from the foot when cutting. This may be a time to use the soapy water as a means to slide the foot free. If an opening to start the saw cannot be found, use the chisel and machinist hammer or Schild panel cutter to start a slot for the saw blade.

Dropping the Sides

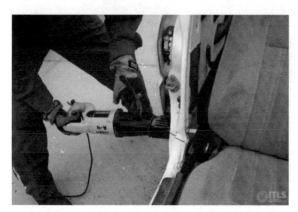

Fig. 126 Relief cut at the bottom of a "B" pillar.

After the roof has been removed, it may be prudent to drop the entire side or sides of the vehicle.

By notching the bottom of the "B" pillar front and back (Fig. 126) and then slipping the long pinch bar into the top of the pillar with the round side down, enough leverage can be applied to take the side to the ground (Fig. 127).

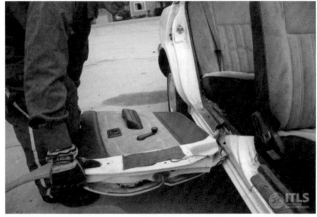

Fig. 127 Use of leverage to push the door toward the ground.

This can be accomplished with the doors still attached by simply cutting the hinges on the front door and unlatching the rear door. This is the reason to cut the "B" pillars high when removing the roof to provide a strength and leverage advantage with a longer "B" pillar.

Work the pinch bar down into the pillar and pull very easy until the back of the "B" pillar. It will tear apart where it is notched.

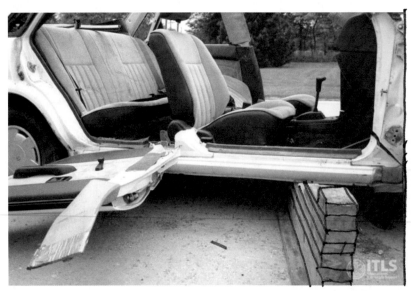

Fig. 128 Sides of car completely dropped.

The entire interior of the vehicle has now been exposed (Fig. 128). The ease of assessment, intervention and packaging has been increased one hundred fold.

Car on Its Wheels — Victim Underneath

In the case of a "backyard mechanic" found underneath the vehicle (Fig. 129), a different approach must be used.

Chock the vehicle as before. Build box cribs on the side away from the victim's head (opposite the side where the victim will be removed). Lift the side slightly to slide cribbing under the vehicle. Move to the other side of the vehicle and with the Hi-Lift Jack

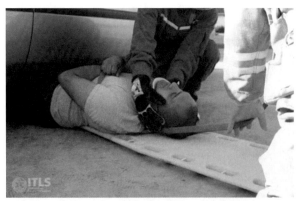

Fig. 129 Use of webbing for mechanical advantage to place the freed victim onto the backboard.

under one wheel well and a bumper jack under the other (same side), jack the vehicle in unison very slowly, cribbing up tight during the maneuver until the victim is free.

Check the far side to make sure the vehicle is not sliding off the cribbing. Never flatten the tires when a victim is under the vehicle.

Key Points to Remember

- It should be stressed that the first job is to get the rescuer to the victim. The second job is to assess the victim and decide whether extrication must be "quick and dirty" or may be done carefully, taking more time. The third job is to extricate the victim.

- Protect victims at all times when cutting.

- Do not pull the steering column:
    - o   It is dangerous.
    - o   It is unnecessary.
    - o   It takes too long.

- Always be aware that tools and jacks can slip. Place them carefully.

- If an inch is needed, do not go two inches!

- Cutting the "B" pillars high gives more leverage when dropping the side.

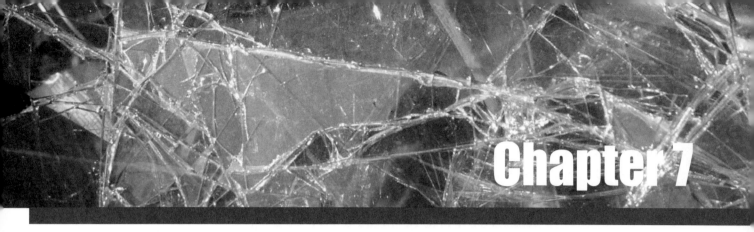

Chapter 7

Packaging & Transfer

Knowledge Objectives

The rescuer should be able to...

- Describe the packaging procedure
- Describe the use of a long spine board and straps or rope sling in three different situations

Skill Objectives

The rescuer should be able to...

- Package the victim for removal
- Use the long spine board and straps or rope sling to remove a victim lying on the front seat of the vehicle
- Use the long spine board and straps or rope sling to remove a victim from the floor behind the front seat
- Use the long spine board and straps or rope sling to remove a victim from underneath a vehicle

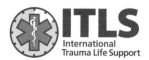

ITLS
International
Trauma Life Support

PACKAGING & TRANSFER

If a spinal injury is suspected, the entire assessment is completed before full spinal motion restrictions since it will not be possible once the victim is secured to the spine board.

Packaging begins once the victim is free from entrapment and terminates when the victim is ready to be removed from the wreckage.

For victims in critical condition, treatment of non-life- or limb-threatening injuries should be delayed until after transport begins.

Remember to remove any and all items that are bulky, sharp or in any way could harm the victim or interfere with securing the victim to the spine board.

Removing an victim involves much more than simply lifting and pulling the victim from the wreckage. It must be accomplished in such a way that existing injuries are not aggravated and new ones are not produced. This is why the prior chapters dealt with creating working space and means of access and exit.

Victims can be removed from an upright vehicle in a number of ways.

An immobilized seated person can be removed through the adjacent door opening on a long spine board. A person who is lying on a seat can be removed on a long spine board or a scoop stretcher. A person who is on the floor of the vehicle can be pulled onto a long spine board with straps or a rope sling.

Victims can be removed from a vehicle that is on its side with a long spine board and straps or a rope sling. Victims who are piled on top of one another can be removed one at a time from the top down.

The use of the long board and straps or rope sling works well in removing a victim from underneath a vehicle that is on its wheels, such as the case of a car slipping off a jack and pinning the victim.

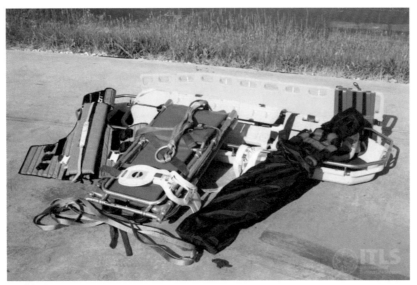

Fig. 130 Equipment used during packaging.

Regardless of the manner of removal from a vehicle, the victim(s) must be firmly secured to a rigid patient carrying device as soon as they are clear of the wreckage.

Long backboards, short backboards, K.E.D.s, M.E.D.s, Sherman vests, scoop stretchers and other such equipment are tools of the trade. Yet, few units employ the long board and rope sling (Fig. 130). The rope sling provides a controlled pull or movement that allows two rescuers to move an injured victim with the least amount of manipulation to the potential C-spine injury.

Removing a Victim Lying on a Vehicle's Seat

When a victim is lying on a vehicle's seat, he or she can be pulled onto a long spine board with a minimum of spinal movement.

A. Have one rescuer get into a position to apply the cervical collar while another rescuer supports the victim's head.

B. Put the victim in as anatomically straight a position as possible, keeping the nose, neck, and navel aligned (Fig. 131).

C. Have one rescuer support the victim's head and shoulders (in a slightly elevated position).

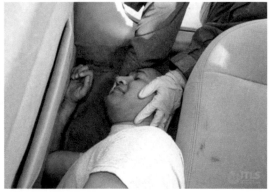
Fig. 131 Attempt to keep the victim's c-spine in the neutral position at all times.

D. Then, slide one end of the spine board between the victim and the seat. Advance the board only to the point where the edge is beyond the shoulder blades (Fig. 132).

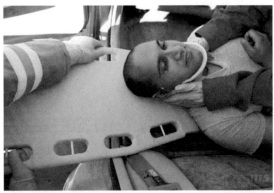
Fig. 132 Place the backboard just past the shoulder blades before sliding the victim into position.

E. Lay the rope sling on the victim's chest at the level of the armpits.

F. Work the sling under the victim's arms so the rope is snug in the armpits (Fig. 133).

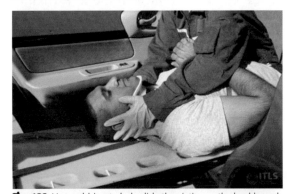
Fig. 133 Use webbing to help slide the victim up the backboard.

G. Slide the adjustment ring behind the cervical collar so that the parallel parts of the sling will help support the victim's head while being pulled onto the board (Fig. 134).

H. Secure the victim's hands together on the abdomen with a Velcro strap, a cravat, or a few turns of cling. This will prevent the arms from moving when pulling on the sling (Fig. 135).

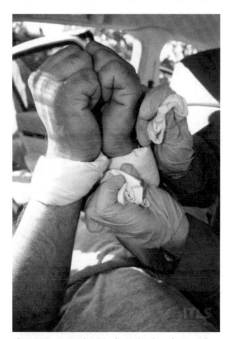
Fig. 135 Consider binding the hands together during movement of the victim.

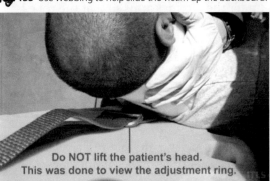
Do NOT lift the patient's head. This was done to view the adjustment ring.
Fig. 134 A slide ring is used to keep webbing in place.

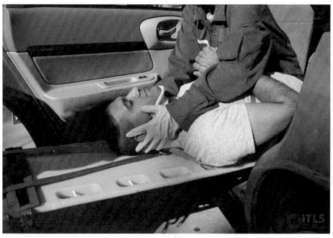 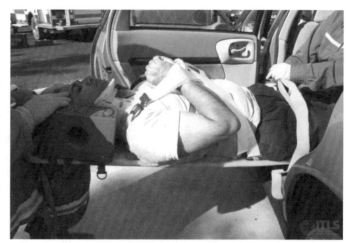

Fig. 136-137 Moving the victim from the vehicle to the backboard.

I. While one rescuer holds the victim in position, move to the end of the board.

J. Exert a smooth, steady pull on the sling to move the victim onto the spine board.

K. Stay as close to the board as possible to prevent lifting the victim's shoulders from the board (Fig. 136-137).

Removing a Victim From the Floor Behind the Front Seat

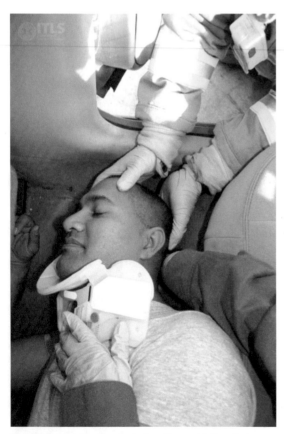

A. Apply a cervical collar (Fig. 138) and with the help of another rescuer, remove the rear seat. Most rear seats are easily removed by pushing down on each side while exerting rearward pressure. Get the seat out of the vehicle. If the seat will not come out in the conventional method, do not waste time trying to outsmart it. Move on.

B. While straddling the victim and supporting the head and shoulders, have another rescuer slide the long spine board under the victim far enough that it is beyond the victim's shoulder blades (Refer back to Fig. 132).

C. While another rescuer holds the board in position, lay the splice over the victim's chest at the level of the armpits.

D. Work the sling under the victim's arms so that the rope is snug in the armpits (Refer back to Fig. 133).

E. Slide the adjustment ring along the rope toward the victim's head and position it under the collar (Refer back to Fig. 134).

F. Secure the victim's hands (Refer back to Fig. 135).

G. While supporting the victim, have another rescuer slowly pull the rope. It may be necessary to raise the victim's legs slightly.

Fig. 138 Applying the cervical motion restriction device.

H. Pull the victim onto the board, staying as close to the board as possible. The adjustment ring will tighten up, thus supporting the victim's head (Refer back to Fig. 137).

I. Secure the victim to the board and transfer.

Removing a Victim From Underneath a Vehicle

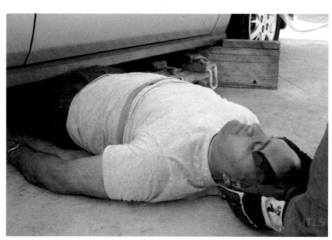

Fig. 139 Until the victim is fully immobilized, continue to stabilize the cervical spine.

The side of the car opposite the victim's head is chocked and cribbed. The egress side is then lifted and cribbed. This method prevents the opposite side from pinning the victim while lifting the head side. The victim should be placed in a cervical collar (Fig. 139).

Make sure there are no penetrating wounds or impaled objects in the chest or abdomen.

If the victim has a back injury or rib or extremity fractures, pulling by the arms, shoulders or clothing is likely to aggravate those injuries.

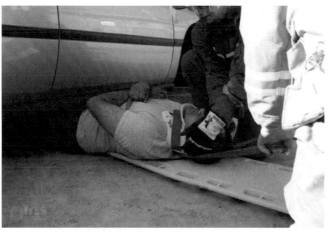

Fig. 140 While your partner is stabilizing the cervical spine, slide the backboard under the victim's shoulder blades.

Using a rope sling to pull the victim onto a long board will involve minimal movement of body parts.

A. Lay the long spine board between two rescuers and close to the victim's head.

B. While one rescuer supports the victim's head, neck and shoulders, slide the board under the victim's shoulder blades (Fig. 140).

C. Gently lower the victim to the board and lay the rope sling on the victim's chest at the level of the armpits.

D. Work the sling under the arms so that the rope is snug in the armpits (Fig. 141).

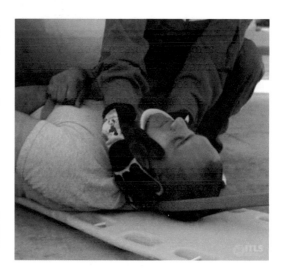

Fig. 141 Position the webbing underneath the victim's arms and across the chest.

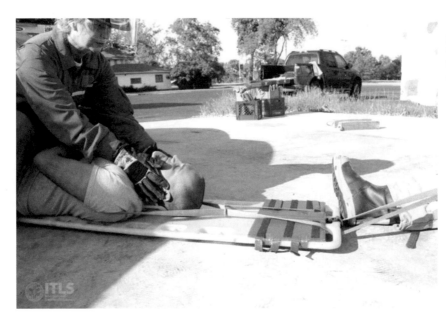

Fig. 142 After adjusting the slide ring, place your webbing through the ends of the backboard.

E. Slide the adjustment ring along the sling until it is under the cervical collar supporting the victim's head (Fig. 142).

F. Kneel at the end of the board and pull slowly. This position will allow the sling to remain flat against the board (Fig. 143).

G. Secure the victim to the board and transfer.

Fig. 143 Continue to maintain cervical spine control until the victim has been fully immobilized.

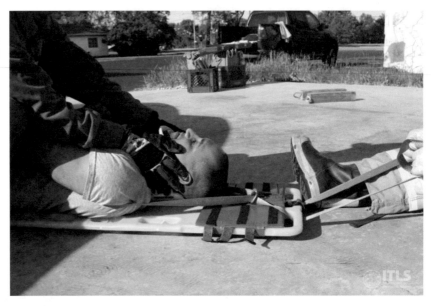

Key Points to Remember

- The goal of spinal motion restriction is to keep the spine in line.

- Align the "Nose - Neck - Navel."

- Move the victim along the "long axis," if not on a board.

- Always secure the victim to a spine board:
    o   With straps securing torso and legs
    o   With a head immobilizer